Dance Meditation
and Zen for the
Black Cancer Patient

Dance Meditation and Zen for the Black Cancer Patient

CARLA STALLING WALTER

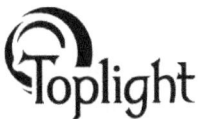

Toplight

Jefferson, North Carolina

ISBN (print) 978-1-4766-9734-5
ISBN (ebook) 978-1-4766-5591-8

LIBRARY OF CONGRESS CATALOGING DATA ARE AVAILABLE

Library of Congress Control Number 2025031019

Front cover images: Shutterstock AI Generator;
background © Numstocker/ Marc Andreu.

Printed in the United States of America

Toplight is an imprint of McFarland & Company, Inc., Publishers

Toplight

Box 611, Jefferson, North Carolina 28640
www.toplightbooks.com

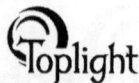

*For Jiryu Rutschman-Byler, my teacher and friend,
Green Dragon Temple Abbot; and all Buddhas and
Ancestors in the Triple World, in the Ten Directions*

Acknowledgments

Several Dharma friends read drafts of this book and provided helpful and insightful comments and suggestions. Appreciation is extended to each of them for their valuable time and freely given efforts to help all beings. In particular, one is my teacher, Jiryu Rutschman-Byler, the abbot at Green Dragon Temple, one of the monasteries with the San Francisco Zen Center. Another is my Dharma Brother Eli Brown-Stevenson, director of inclusion and belonging with the San Francisco Zen Center.

I'd also like to thank my husband.

It wouldn't be possible for this book to co-arise dependently in this space if it wasn't for my birth parents, and all those who serve as Great Teachers along this path from beginningless time. Gratitude is extended to those beings, too.

Table of Contents

Preface

What are the teachings of a whole lifetime? An appropri-
ate statement.—Ch'ung-hsien 2006, p. 86

In this preface, I share with you, hoping to show you a sense of my small life, who I am and why I wrote this book for you. My purpose in putting this here now is to provide a background into, or insight about, my experiences, which have led me to embrace the practice of Zen and Dance Meditation and their Dharmas. It would be good if you read this section before you begin the rest of the book. I know I often skip this part of books, thinking I'd like to get to the point, and might come back to it later.

Background Scenes

Leaning on cars in the street was a thing we did. Cars represented wealth and status in the community. People stood around outside and had conversations leaning on cars, opened the doors and blared music out into the street; men drank and told jokes; children played double–Dutch or stickball; women gossiped and hung out. It's what we did.

One afternoon I leaned on a car across the street from the junior high with the neighborhood American Black teenagers, laughing, having fun joking around, smoking cigarettes. Tisha Ferguson shouted, "Get off the car, Carla." She was a mean girl, and in the seventh grade had already gotten the rep of being a bit promiscuous. In the locker room after our gymnastics meets, she walked around naked, spewing nasty words as she gyrated. One time, Coach Miss

Jackson came out and told her to get dressed and go to the office. Tisha said, towering over the coach, right up in her face, "Make me." All the girls gasped! You didn't mess with Miss Jackson. Ferguson didn't flinch. Jackson pivoted and walked over to the intercom and called security.

Now Anita McRae, the other proudly self-proclaimed love to love who went to church and justified her going with whomever was the current jock in her stories, singing Earth, Wind & Fire songs as she did, was also watching along with all the other thirty girls. My being the four-eyed bookworm with straight A's introduced another level of difference between us.

Then Ferguson said, "What-you looking at, Carla?" as the guard moved her along, and she was then wrapped in a white towel. Looking and seeing directly was disrespectful in the Black community. We turned our stares away from domestic violence bruises and fights, people's clothes thrown in the street, men standing on the corner, for example. Ferguson beat people up after school. Just looking at her could be a cause for her rage. So far, I'd avoided fighting her and others, and that was very skillful. Look, in elementary school I kicked some serious butt once or twice when the girls wouldn't stop the harassment, so I had no choice.

When Ferguson ordered me off the car, I stood up and backed away and went to lean on another car. I burned with the feeling of powerlessness, though I didn't want to fight.

And then, last year, at a board meeting I was chairing, Yelandha, an American Black city councilwoman, said to me, "I'm warning you, don't you be talking to the people over at the county. You don't know what you doing and you don't know the history. I'm telling you, you better come through me first. Don't burn no bridges before you even get started." She's a mean girl, too, except now she's a middle-aged, educated, early retired sorority sister person. Yelandha complains about people misspelling her name if they spell it *Yolanda*, boasts and brags about sitting on important boards and the city council, where she expounds, to anyone who will listen, how much power she has, through the lens of Black cultural resistance and entitlement. Only she actually is all lip and doesn't keep promises; everyone knows that so they just nod as she talks.

When Yelandha told me not to talk to people, for a split second, I felt that powerlessness that I felt back in the seventh grade, as if I was going to suffer harm if I didn't do what she commanded. Or that another human being had power over me. At the moment turning within, seeing her as a suffering person who needed compassion, seeing her conditioning as a Black woman from the south, breathing in Zazen as I'd learned to do, sitting there at the table with eleven other people, all Black except for two, fear disappeared. I realized she and I weren't separate—we were simply here together. She wasn't an object, outside of me. There was nothing to gain from her, nothing to prove. Nothing to resist or fight. I just moved the board on to the next topic. My feelings of powerlessness evaporated.

Not too long ago I was on the phone with my mother. She was telling me about her upcoming trip to Kansas City, going there with my older sister, so my sister could attend an annual conference. There was a time—for many decades—when I felt jealous of these adventures or excursions with the two of them. With wisdom, it occurred to me to remind her that I'd lived in the Kansas City area for several years. And she remembered that I'd invited her there once or twice and the good time she had. At that juncture I was able to feel true joy for her and my sister, as well as compassion for them both.

Now, don't get me wrong. They both complain to me about each other when the other one's not around, and, according to what they said to me, neither of them wanted to go with the other on this trip. My mother needed to take the trip since she was experiencing cabin fever, having moved from southern California to Asheville, North Carolina, a couple of years ago. My sister needed to bring my mother with her to assuage the fear of leaving her alone, knowing my mother's ailments.

My mother, an American Black woman, is a product of culture and antiblack racism, being born during the Depression Era and raised in Oklahoma. My father—part Cuban, part American Black, born in 1928—was shot dead in a strip mall by police officers in Los Angeles when I was twelve over a pair of $1 earrings. Later, when I was an adult and had a chance to read the autopsy report, I learned that his blood alcohol was at a poisonous level, and the police report stated that he started shooting first. Who knows whether the records are true or not? Only what is true is that he died just like many American Black men and other men of color do these days: for seemingly ridiculous and petty reasons. And I have to point out, some are killed by American Black police officers, too. Anyway, of course, no doubt my sister and I are also products of the antiblack cultural superstructure. My family isn't unique.

So, there's a lot of suffering, and individual and collective causes and conditions that foster repeated behaviors driven by greed, anger, and delusion. Or we can say, wanting, protecting, and being unaware of how situations can drive us without our knowing it.

I said culture *and* antiblack racism. You know what I'm talking about. It's the norms of the American culture and the expectations put on us through it *and* the way antiblack racism tears and shatters both the culture we grow up in and our dreams and hopes developed within it. This equally applies to American Latins, Middle Easterners, Africans, Asians, and anyone who is marginalized due to skin color or other difference.

I was born in south central Los Angeles. I identify as an American Black woman, the gender I was born with. Not too long after my father was killed, I made up my mind to get out of that environment, not to blame the system, and not to be bitter. In order to make a different life for myself, I left the city altogether. I personally paid for, with the help of grants and loans, and earned bachelor's, master's, and doctoral degrees from public research universities. I taught in and I also successfully led higher education institutions with few, if any, people of color, let alone American Blacks. I've also led private organizations in which I was the only Black person working there. For many years, I tried to ignore the impact that antiblack racism had on me. In my career, I set my mind on not being poor. I acknowledged my childhood culture, while I didn't let it be in the forefront of my decisions and behaviors. Today I embrace all of these causes and conditions and draw upon the practice of Dance and Zen Buddhist meditation to provide compassion and help others. In these pages, I share with you what I've learned about how the self and its ego are sources of suffering for people of color, and about releasing ourselves and others from it through Zen Buddhism.

My Spiraling Road of Spiritual Practices

Even though it exists, as a child I was not consciously aware of "Buddha Nature."

In my neighborhood gang members were hating, killing, stealing, lying, and selling and pushing drugs. Many neighbors, though, were employed in stable pensionable places and wanted the best education for their children, as well as a peaceful, financially secure life. Only due to segregation and historical antiblack racism, and even after desegregation, we lived in community with the gangs. As a source of ease and hope, the Black church was a bedrock for many, and it had become that when slaves turned to it rather than try to keep their home country's practices, and owing to the fact that they were excluded from the white churches.

When I was a child, many went to church each week where we heard emotionally charged sermons reinforcing or producing their beliefs of "the system" being the barrier to happiness and the creator of disdain for Blacks. The pastors encouraged all to call on Jesus, and to look to the next life for bliss and redress. During my life I've studied and practiced Christianity. I served as a deaconess, an usher, and committed to upholding the Old and New Testaments. The issues that troubled me in adhering to Christianity were mainly around the way the Bible was interpreted and the external locus of control for salvation.

Eventually I set the church aside, seeking other ways, ways that didn't necessarily keep antiblack racism stable, and that answered more of my questions on death and what happens to human beings. Being hesitant for so long, as I heard so many admonishments about looking outside the church, it took a while. Some said I'd be changed into something evil if I went to the movies. Others said I'd be worshiping idols if I went to another religion. Some said I'll surely go to the devil's place if I break loyalty to the church. And some said dance was the devil's domain. I found all of these to be pure threats with no substance. Nothing happened when I went to the movies. There were no different circumstances in my life that arose as a result of leaving the church. And I certainly didn't experience anything like idol worship or wind up in a bad place arising from dancing.

Anyway, I studied the Kabbalah extensively and mystical Judaism and found it somewhat more reasonable in answering the question of humans relative to the larger universe. I was also following a path set out by Eknath Easwaran (1993), who advocated that all religions have something to offer, and his program of passage meditation. In that, one memorized a passage from a religion, such as Psalm 23 or the Prayer of Saint Francis of Assisi. This was the anchor for meditation, which he advocated doing for twenty minutes a day. He also said we need a mantra, some kind of phrase to repeat as we go through the day, so that when the mind goes on in directions drumming up anxiety and fear, there's an alternative to focus on. People could choose their own mantras from their religions, such as *I can do all things through Christ who strengthens me.* Or one could repeat the name of God that is applicable to their religion.

While I was exploring different spiritual paths, I, like many others, bumped up against a whole world of corporations selling me the path to attaining happiness. I call it the mindfulness marketplace. It's a billion-dollar industry.

In that marketplace, I found one path that promised I'd be able to manifest what I wanted. It states that I have what I have, that is, lack of stuff, money, happiness, success, and so on, is arising from what I think. Now this is a sort of Buddhist idea too, in the sense that it's the mind that supports the self. For certain, Buddhists don't say your mind is the reason for your not having millions of dollars and the so-called sweet life of the wealthy. In Buddhism, we see that the cause of suffering is desire. Increasing desires and trying to constantly fulfill them heads us in an unsatiable direction.

The mindfulness marketplace is where people are being sold all kinds of consumer goods to help them. You can find apps offering classes and retreats and sermons and gurus. Certifications. Crystals, beads, and smells. Books, spas, body cleanses and mind-altering sweat lodges. And this list is a short one! True, some arouse the true awakening for enlightenment in myriad ways, including while wandering in this marketplace. Like nearly all thriving enterprises, the mindfulness marketplace exists owing to people needing something to make them feel better, to help them with their fears, anxieties, desires, feelings of being separate, and questions about their lives. And the mindfulness market makes promises that you'll be calmer, have better relationships, and in some cases have more wealth and better health.

It's not so much that it's unskillful to have these. It's just that the attainment of what is promised is based on self, on ego, on looking at what others have, on greed. Following this logic, you can't get out of the cycle of wanting, so to speak, since grasping for what's promised is empty. It's never enough. Another mindfulness product is positioned as meditation. You can find many kinds, and you can also get apps to help you with this. Though not all Buddhist practices are concerned with profit taking, different schools of Buddhism have varied approaches to meditation. In the chapters of this book, I'm going to focus on Zen Buddhism. Other schools of Buddhism are out there, such as Rinzai, Theravadan, Nichiren, Tibetan, and plenty more, depending on location and histories. My focus doesn't allow me to cover all of these. I encourage you to inquire into them so you can understand any nuances for yourself.

What's Zen Buddhism?

As I said, there are multiple paths of Buddhism and each person has to decide what's best for them. I've done research and reading, continuing to now as well, and I concluded that Zen Buddhism is right for me, seeing the way it presents practice, ethics, morality, and explores and explains psychological aspects of the mind. The latter point is important to changing our thinking and developing a way out of the mind's conditioning in racism. Zen Buddhism has a long history and incorporates aspects of historical Buddhism.

Importantly, in Zen meditation, called Zazen, practitioners sit with their eyes open, facing a wall, focusing on the breath while stilling the thoughts. Another main and very important aspect is that Zen Buddhism proposes that enlightenment is right here. You don't have to earn it. Further, your aspiration for peace is the aspiration for enlightenment. It can happen in a split second, today and tomorrow, or continuously.

In Zen Buddhism, there is a movement called "Kinhin" which I will come back to later in the book, along with some other movements incorporated into the practice. I'm a firm believer that dance movement and realization of Buddha Mind are one within nondiscursiveness, and this can aid in staying attentive throughout life, day to day. I use the word "attentive" purposely so that it doesn't get manipulated within other discourses that don't serve us. Attentive means to be in the present moment, without concern with or obsession with self.

My Encounter with Zen Buddhism

On a chance visit to Tassajara Zen Monastery (Tassajara from now on) with my sister, the first thing I encountered was no Internet, no cell coverage. In the first day or so, I felt weird, as if the world was gone; there was no way to check the weather, see email, make a call, or search for anything. You could wait in line to use the only landline telephone on the property. Since my sister was there, the one I told you about earlier who was driving to Kansas City with my mother, I felt some ease.

Tassajara is in the Big Sur Mountains above Carmel Valley, California. There's nothing nearby, other than more mountains. Getting from the bottom of the mountain up to the monastery requires a sturdy four-wheel-drive vehicle and a strong stomach. Some take motion sickness pills before they travel the road; it's windy and full of deep gouges, and goes alongside the mountain's switchbacks, showing sheer cliff dropoffs on one side.

Tassajara's summer guest season is what we were attending.

Workshops, retreats, programs—and a bookstore to support all of that. People flock there thanks to the solitude and the detachment from the workaday frenzied world of texts, calls, social media, emails, you get my point. People want to let go of that constant pull for them to be "on." You get to let go very deeply at Tassajara.

Tassajara has another claim to fame: food! Guests receive fully vegetarian meals prepared by excellent chefs. The food is wonderful. You can get Tassajara cookbooks if you'd like to try a few recipes (Brown, 2011). I was a vegetarian long before taking the Zen Buddhist Precepts; it was the meals during our retreat that reinforced my resolve to try new recipes. They provide ease in following the vow we take not to kill.

We stayed at Tassajara for a week. It was really hot during the month of August. At night, my sister and I lay outside and gazed at the millions of stars, which we'd never seen before. In the lights of the city of course, you maybe see one or two, a few stars. Wow, it was amazing how dark it was. Then one day we went to Zazen instruction, and I sat my first Zazen the next morning. When I got back home, I started going to San Francisco Zen Center on Saturdays for their Zazen and Dharma talk program. Dharma talks are talks given by Dharma teachers with a message of some sort, and I went to them regularly. I also listened to them via podcasts or archives or attended them online. I began sitting Zazen every morning before leaving the house. Eventually I made my way to another monastery of the San Francisco Zen Center, Green Dragon Temple in Marin County, California. That's where I met my teacher. Today, I'm a lay Zen Buddhist practitioner, via that long winding religious path I outlined above. I have taken the Precepts, which means that I vowed to uphold the practices of Zen Buddhism and to help people in their lives. I practice with the San Francisco Zen Center and the Chapel Hill Zen Center.

Different kinds of sitting periods aside from the daily practice are offered. After a while I went to what's known as a half-day retreat, then a one-day, then a three-day retreat. Then, I was able to go to what's called *Rohastu* to celebrate Buddha's Enlightenment. It's a seven-day retreat. That was fantastic for me; resting on the virtue of the shorter retreats, I received Zazen sitting into my body and mind, like a muscle memory. At the longer retreats, I was able to see my ego very clearly. Then I began to question everything and unthink some of my judgments and see how I keep myself enmeshed with my own suffering. Like, I had a lot of preconceived ideas so that when they weren't manifested, I got angry or felt jealous or got depressed. Over time, I read books by Shunryu Suzuki Roshi, the founder of the San Francisco Zen Center, and other Zen Buddhist teachers. They helped me see where my anger, jealousy, and disappointments were types of greed, hate or anger, and delusion. These kept me "stuck" in pain, and a lot of it was from beliefs I held about being an American Black and living the cultural conditioning it provides. I had to learn to address the thoughts and then let them go in order to see that I'm always the subject and everything else the object in my little mind's eye.

Diagnosed with Multiple Myeloma

During this time, I continued Dance Dharma, even though I had a very stressful and demanding career in higher education. So when I received an unbelievable, out-of-the-blue and nearly accidental life-threatening, advanced-stage diagnosis of multiple myeloma (MM from now on), I was totally floored. MM is a bone-marrow cancer that crowds out healthy cells, attacking the bones and blood. I had already established a spiritual practice. Be sure, even if you have not started practicing, you can start at any time before, during, or after a cancer or other diagnosis.

Along with having Zen Buddhism arise in my life through many turnings and gates, I've always found peace in dance. Since I was a young child, I've been intrigued by dance and spiritual practices. For a good part of my life just as with spiritual practice, I have been involved with dance, either teaching, studying, performing, or writing about it, while at the same time engaging the pathway of spiritual practice. When I was presented with the opportunity to attend a doctoral program, I was undecided between entering religious studies or dance history and theory programs. I chose the dance program because it seemed to allow an encompassing of both dance and religion. During the time I was in graduate school, and in fact in the experiences I had with dance before and after it, I solidified for myself that dance is both indigenous and social, and nondiscursive. That is, dance can communicate without words and before meanings are attached and should not be judged good or bad. This perfectly fits with positioning dance as meditation and spiritual practice in line with Dance Dharma.

Though my first career was finance oriented, not knowing at the time about Right Livelihood, which I talk about in Chapter 2, with an epiphany and opportunity, I chose dance history and theory as my doctoral program. At that time, I had become disillusioned with the cultural conditions dictating that I need to have a business career. Therefore, I have done research and written a lot about dance and am still writing about it. During my business career and after it, I taught, choreographed, and performed dance, particularly ballet, and later, sacred dance as my avocation. My experiences with dance were part and parcel to my realizing this practice path and being able to stay attentive in my life.

In 2022 with that MM diagnosis, my Zen and dance practice played a large part of bringing about my healing and recovery. I feel like I've been led to share Zen Buddhism and Dance Dharma with you, raising awareness around the way American Blacks and some people of color are treated in the health care system. My recent experience has given me the focus needed to do my best to navigate it. Poor or substandard care in the United States has been and is a very long road rife with exclusionary difference.

I want you to have freedom from what the Buddha called greed (wanting and desire), hate (anger), and delusion (confusion), so that you can see the way out of suffering, and bring others with you through practicing Zazen. I also want you to know about Dance Dharma, how it shows up in practice, and how it can shape realization of reality. All I ask is that you keep an open mind as you go on this journey.

An Opening

If we can sit upright in this field of suffering, letting the deities of the subconscious come and go, then our stillness becomes the antidote to the greed, hate, and delusion that are the source of our torment.—The Third Turning of the Wheel (Anderson, 2012, p. 69)

Even though Buddhism has a long, meandering history dating to the early third century BCE (Lopez, 2009), it's proposed that Zen Buddhism arrived in California in the United States around 1850 through Chinese immigrants taking advantage of the Gold Rush: Chinese immigrants who established practice centers, some in San Francisco and some in Hawaii, until they were forced out of the United States by the government in 1854, due to the claim that they were taking jobs away from Americans (Wikipedia, n.d., "Timeline of Zen Buddhism in the United States"). At the same time, Japan was turned to as an exchange partner for the United States for goods and services. Americans discriminated against the Chinese violently, harming their businesses and excluding them from working in the country. The Chinese Exclusion Act disallowed Chinese people from working in or returning to the United States. The immigrants experienced lynching through the 1880s to the mid–1900s. Around this time, the United States showed preference for Japanese immigrants. In 1906 the United States called for separate but equal schools of Asians and Asian immigrants. By 1924, the Asian Exclusion Act was passed to keep Asians out of the United States and to deny them citizenship. During 1942, Japanese internment happened, putting Japanese people in concentration camps. In 1965, the Asian Exclusion Act was rescinded.

Dance Meditation and Zen for the Black Cancer Patient

Many of us know the history of African slavery in the West, the taking of lands from First Nations peoples, and the traumatic mark it has left on the psyche, the deep consciousnesses of people of all ethnicities. Each of these unwholesome acts was rooted in greed, hate, and delusion, and in many instances was paired with missionary work and Christianity. Such a pairing created a complicit mindset among some Africans and American Black people. Antiblack racism was the learned, tested, and proven discriminatory platform on which those from China and Japan were treated. We also know that racism and bigotry continue as you read these words.

Nevertheless, by 1903 Japanese Soto Zen was established in Hawaii and it moved through the United States from that point, beginning in San Francisco and moving eastward. From around the 1950s Soto Zen Buddhism grew through white Americans taking up the practice, particularly in response to the wars and the unrests in Civil Rights taking place in the 1960s and 1970s (see *Buddhism in America Timeline*, as well as the Wikipedia entry). The first American Black woman that received Dharma transmission, or recognition as a successor of the Buddha in this lineage, was Merle Kodo Boyd in 2006. What's that—more than a century from when Soto Zen was established? That same year, for the first time an American Black male, Jules Shuzen Harris, received it as well. Osho Zenju Earthlyn Manuel is also an American Black woman receiving Dharma transmission in 2016 in the Suzuki Roshi Soto Zen lineage, which is the organization that I'm associating with. angel Kyodo williams (the lettering case is hers) is the second American Black woman to become a fully ordained and Dharma transmitted Soto Zen priest, in 2013, through the Zen Peacemaker Order and White Plum lineage of the Soto Zen tradition. My point is that it's taken a while for Soto Zen Buddhism to reach American Blacks, and for Asian Americans to be allowed here. I'm grateful that both have taken place.

Embedded in American history is substandard, and/or nonexistent, and/or nonconsensual experimental medical treatment of American Blacks and other people of color. It was not until 1868 that we were individually considered a whole human being. Even so, terrible treatment within the dominant health care system continued for decades, and still impacts treatment choices for today's illnesses, childbearing, and diseases.

When people see me, a brown-skin woman, no matter their ethnicity or race, generally they make racial assumptions and projections. I do it, too, and we human beings in the United States can't help it considering it's a conditioned response. During COVID, many displays of racism were shown on screens around the world, to some viewers' "surprise." At the same time, seeing those visceral displays, many white people engaged in studying their roles in keeping antiblack racism and its negative impacts alive and how they could change their beliefs and behaviors. So in addition to the importance of Zen and Dance Meditation while in medical therapy for cancer, and the efficacy of only taking appropriate medicines, I want to talk about how Black people stabilize antiblack racism as unknown to them just as often as MM is to many. I give some ideas of how our beliefs and behaviors may change by practicing Zen Buddhism, and how these changes in perspectives aid in sustaining and expanding health: mentally, emotionally, and physically.

Who This Book Is For

As I wrote, I thought of and visualized American BIPOCs who have some experience with living disappointments, suffering, greed, hate, and delusion from antiblack racism. This book is for those who have experienced racism in its many flavors and those who also perpetuate bigotry and difference among the BIPOC groups. As a result of being born in the United States, or having lived here for a while, the antiblack racism touches you, influences you in such a way as you see others with the clouded messages to drive separation and difference. It might make you think that, as Arsenio Hall might have said, "Those BIPOC people over there are the problem, I'm not." BIPOCs can benefit greatly from this book in that it delves into the mind and thinking, how we are products of cultural causes and conditioning that we often perpetuate. The book is also for BIPOC people who practice Zen Buddhism, and for those who teach that it's only the white people who need to change. We all must change by looking deeply at our egos and self-based propulsions. The goal is to release ourselves from attachments to beliefs and behaviors, and to discern what is real.

When I was diagnosed with MM, I had never faced my death in a real way. I understood the concept of impermanence by experiencing several people in my family having died when I was very young. No one talked to me about their deaths though. No one spoke of grief or grieving.

The diagnosis moment forced me to look at death and what it means. In our Western culture we don't deal with death directly. And at least for me, I was unprepared for what my mind and emotions did, bringing up pains and mistakes from as far back as I could remember, causing deep personal suffering in addition to the terminal diagnosis.

We see death on television or experience it when loved ones or people we know die. These aren't the live cultural aspects, generally, where we see dead people for real or talk about what goes on inside the mind. We don't want to touch a dead body, be near a corpse, or live in a place where someone has died recently. Truly when we do consider it, we might fantasize about death, abstractly thinking we'll die in a car crash or airplane mishap. Sadness surrounds death too, along with a good deal of misunderstanding about what death is. We're told in Christianity: heaven, or hell, it's up to you. My Buddhist practice helped me go through the confusion arising from a diagnosis of terminal cancer and come out of it with a clearer perspective on death and dying.

While in treatment I was offered emotional support via a therapist, which was great. That helped in many ways. More actively, with my lifelong experience with dance meditation, during the depths of fatigue and sadness, I indirectly engaged with emotional imbalance. It's been shown that dance as an adjuvant therapy helps with slowing disease progression, physically, mentally, and emotionally. In fact there are dance movement therapists trained in this. That's wonderful. People in cancer and other treatments can avail themselves of dance meditation without a dance therapist too.

The book is therefore not only for BIPOC folks receiving cancer treatments; it casts a wide net that includes doctors, dance movement therapists, nurses, chaplains, and others in treatment centers and hospitals who deal with American Blacks and other people of color with cancer. I also invite those working in hospice care to read and internalize the contents of this book. For those in the medical field, it's critical to understand how to offer support to the treatment and the dying process beyond the medicinal protocols and the mainstream Christian view of life and death, and to know the history that has undermined health and well-being for marginalized and poor people.

Since I have experience with Soto Zen Buddhism first and foremost as a salve for calming my raging and inflamed angry ego relative to racism, and I'm an American Black woman, and lastly as I have been through the trials and difficulties of navigating the dominant health care system, I believe this book is critical for each American Black and person of color to read. It would benefit health care providers and people associated with pharmaceuticals to read as well.

No, I'm not an ordained Buddhist priest. I'm not a doctor or medical professional, nor am I setting myself out as an authority on being an American Black. I don't want to cast stereotypes on any being. It's not my intention to stir up anger over history, nor to deny it or set out to place blame on people who have lived experiences of trajectories of hate or even to explain why it exists. To be clear, rather, my purpose is to offer some solace on dealing with issues that arise in this life in this world where racism and bigotry define our every thought it seems, to offer ways of being that are not only life-changing for you. Vision-changing. Providing a byproduct, for changing community and the general cultural landscape. Erasure of lines and learned thoughts. Ways to take care of yourself inside and outside of the healthcare system. The importance of movement meditation as well as Zazen. What I offer is to share with you the path I followed, a way out of framing some of the causes and conditions that could make for increased illness, greed, hate, and delusion. You'll have to explore these and others you'll find as a result on your own, of course. Why? The Zen Buddhist practice and obtaining decent medical care are not about being told what to do or believe. It requires your own skillful and relentless and continuous inquiry.

An Overview of the Book

In Zen Buddhism I learned that we are shaped by causes and conditions often unknown to us. In the first chapter I attempt to cover some of this ground by talking about how a child experiences cultural norms such as music and dance, food, clothing, domestic violence, addictions, education, work and employment. After that I turn to loyalties that are oftentimes culturally expected, and then to religion. The chapter closes with telling you what Zen Buddhism is and isn't. For the reason that I only have my experience to draw on, I relate it to living in poor neighborhoods, growing up in the 1960s in the inner city, within a family that was plagued by greed, hate and anger, and delusion. I know that not everyone has this experience, and that there are wealthy American BIPOC families. I hope this will not turn you away; instead, my intention would be for you to embrace the fact that racism and bigotry are conditioned and constructed, and they serve to support and validate inequities in every aspect of life. For me, practicing Zen Buddhism with my teacher in the Suzuki Roshi Soto Zen Lineage has given me a new way to look at the world I live in, namely, by seriously examining causes and conditions that structure my ego. The ego is the base, the root, of greed, hate and anger, and delusion. Rather than living by causes and conditions, I live by vow.

The seemingly Westernized human desire for fame and gain, along with dualistic thinking, takes center stage in Chapter 2. Within the chapter I open the doors of my heart and pour out my understanding of the Zen Buddhist notions of self-centeredness couched in deeply rooted self-dislike. From these ways of thinking we ensure that we live within causes and conditions that force suffering to keep happening in our lives and those of our loved ones. A lot of the suffering comes from believing things in this life are permanent. After all, that's not true. Impermanence surrounds us at all times, and especially the impermanence of this life we are living. We grasp for something to hold onto, something to attain or gain that we call "mine," and the grasping results in pain, as it is never fulfilling, at least not for long. At this point I introduce the *Four Noble Truths* and the *Noble Eightfold Path* of the Buddha, then turn to the *Wisdom Paramitas* as the process for reducing suffering. The end of Chapter 2 brings you to a discussion of Zen Buddhism for American Blacks, explaining Buddha Nature that is accessible for you as you embrace the process.

When I get to Chapter 3, I share the power of dance as I experienced it as a meditation practice. I found out that I wasn't alone in this experience, and that in fact it had been going on since people began living on Earth, or at least, a very long time ago. Not only is dance a meditation practice, it also provides well-being aspects for the body and mind. While it's not necessarily obvious, Buddhists have a relationship with dance, too. Many Tibetan Buddhists dance in rituals, for sure, and they also stage dances as a way of making money for their temples and communities. Even so, in Zen Buddhism dance is more subdued. I like to think of the movements in Zen Buddhism as dances even if they aren't called that. In particular, there is a walking meditation, movement that resembles a slow-moving dance, with a body posture and steps, as well as some of what are called "forms" during which the movements are very choreographed and embody a sense of awe. I go into these in some detail in the third chapter. After that, I talk about the Buddha and the Bodhisattva Path, then offer a conversation about birth and death. Here I discuss the meaning of enlightenment as I understand it in Zen Buddhism, establishing a daily practice, and why having a teacher makes for a skillful activity. The chapter isn't meant to give you a full history, only to provide an overview.

In Chapter 4, which begins the second part of the book, my story comes to light. It's a story about my encounter with the health care system when I was diagnosed with MM in early 2023. The chapter includes the ways in which the cancer manifests, and how the medical community looks at it, and the decisions I made to engage with dance meditation (what I call Dance Dharma) and Zazen along with some of the prescriptions suggested for the disease, in order to overcome it. Cancer treatment isn't equitable, and this forms the basis and the heart of the fifth chapter. I get deep into the history of medical treatment for American Blacks and people of color. While it's true that this history is really painful, there are and were American Blacks and people of color with wealth that allowed and supported the social and economic structures within their cultural groups. That means that not every American Black or person of color experiences disparity and neglect. In any event, I try to give you some pointers on how to be assertive in the medical system to look after your own well-being and financial situation, whatever it is. Finally, I give some insight, again based on my experience, to help you with dealing with your quality of life as a person with cancer.

Entering Chapter 6, you'll find an honest discussion on life and death from the Zen Buddhist perspective, again as I understand it today. That is followed by some serious words on setting up a will and trust, and empowering you with beneficial actions dealing with the reality of your birth and death cycle. I next offer words by way of a continued opening process, sharing where I am now in regard to MM. Finally, I leave you with references and places of support for your study, continued wellness, and embodiment of the Soto Zen Buddhist path.

I try to capitalize terms that are used in this practice, such as Zazen, Dance Dharma, Bodhisattva, Buddha Nature, and the like. I hope this will draw you into the importance of the deeper meanings that are contained within them.

For clarity, throughout the book I use capitalized words and italics to denote words and phrases that are important in Zen Buddhism. Also, the phrase "American Black" I define as a person who lives in the United States and has some African heritage. American "person of color" is also understood in this way, leaving aside African lineages. The latter definition applies to people whose families were born here or who immigrated. Together, these are meant to define American BIPOC.

PART ONE

1

Cultural Norms and Conditions

Who You Think You Are

When you think you know the way you don't
Ego prevents intimacy and the opportunity to help others
Both block Buddha Dharma—Tanahashi, 2013, 191

Zen Buddhism, through the lineage of the Buddha, tells us about suffering and then it explains to us how to overcome it. At a minimum, it's about looking at, and noticing, sense perceptions and mental formations—the stories we tell ourselves, why we feel the way we do, the projections we make about this life. It's an aspect of taking time to slow down. Asking yourself why you do what you do. Yes: Meditation. And a whole way of being that can at first seem so foreign from what we're used to. All the same, I've done it, and it's been, for me, a way out of much of my antiblack racial suffering.

Let me bracket this before I start in directly on some aspects and details of Zen Buddhism as I understand it at this moment. I think it's important to lay down some foundation about how Black people, some of us, the majority of us anyway, have been mentally and emotionally habitually programmed to suffer unconsciously over time. I'm talking about cultural norms, or how some of us are shaped by what we're told and how we're treated. What we focus on. And my point of view will be from my American Black experience, which, by the way, isn't monolithic. There is no "one" universal Black experience. A way to think about it instead embraces facets of culture and histories that make up individual and collective interactions. All it takes is a song, a dance, and a plate of food to get me feeling like, remembering, identifying, yes, this is my culture. This is what we do, this is how we do it! Stated in broad terms, the mass of this culture and history are who we are as a collective who have shared histories, shared experiences. Not to worry: I'm not going to spend too much time on this in the interest of moving beyond it. I keep it, don't push it away, while we move beyond it. I'm going to start with how a child is raised, then go on to talk briefly about music, dance, food, clothes and cars, domestic violence, addictions, work, loyalty, and religion. The reason for this is to bring in how our egos and self-orientation drive a belief in who we are. This is true for many cultures, not just Black culture. Next I'll delve into Zen Buddhism and go from there.

As an American Black Child Grows

In our families and communities, culture plays a tremendous part in shaping who we think we are or who we think we should be, or what is, turns out to be, our egos. From early ages, we're socialized with cultural objects and situations that tell us how to behave and think. It starts with children before they're born. Cultural objects and situations adults lay on children include tangible and intangible referents. As the child grows up, they're conditioned to think they're separate from those objects and other people, and this idea of separateness continues into old age for many of us. Unless, of course, we are turned toward an aspiration for enlightenment. That's usually a moment when we experience something that sparks us to seeing there's more to this objective life of suffering.

For children, very familiar tangible objects are clothing, foods, toys, their homes, cars, and these days, electronic devices and educational gadgets. Intangibles reach into how a child experiences events and relationships, how the parents treat the child, what the others in the family or community communicate to the child, and unspoken, projected thinking and opinions on the parts of the family members, television, social media, and people in the child's life. Each communication also includes causes and conditions that shaped the family histories, and the ancestors, and as well, the expectations that are unspoken and saddled on the child for future outcomes. For example, the child may pick up cues that they are going to be successful by carrying on a legacy or be unsuccessful thanks to being like so and so, who was no good. Or they may get subtle communications from television or other media that tells them they need to wear certain kinds of clothes or act certain ways in terms of their sexuality. The reactions demonstrated by their guardians, teachers, and people they look up to also dictate information to the child and form the mind's way of being.

The child hears music, watches people dance, sees people engage in sporting events, maybe goes to church, learns what to wear, what food to like, what to drink, who goes to work and who doesn't, the value of education, who to be loyal to, and what religion or no religion means. They also try to figure out their sexuality and gender. And even though developing humans in the West may go through phases of rejection or acceptance of aspects of these and other cultural practices, they are nevertheless embedded in our consciousness. As we know, some songs, dances, and cultural attire used in commercials can invoke feelings that prompt us into buying things we don't need, helping to us remember products many years later in our lives (McCracken, 1986; Walter, 2012, 2015). Many affinities are developed that form likes and dislikes, preferences if you understand what I'm trying to convey, through these connections. And songs, dances, and clothing themselves activate our senses, thoughts, feelings, and points of view toward each other and often come up as a way of comparing our culture and social standing to those of others, as well as creating differences, feelings of separation, and uncorroborated beliefs that can ultimately cause suffering.

Music and Dance

In my culture, music is a stable source of pleasure, support, and resistance. My parents and family loved Black vocalists, jazz, blues, gospel, and classical music particularly played by American Black orchestras. A lot of Black people's music soothed racist events and reminded people of love, or complained about the same problems. My father also liked music by Neil Young, who often sang about racism's negative impacts. It was fantastic that both my parents really enjoyed the music that allowed escape from the day-to-day life of struggle or that validated their pain, valorized lovemaking. And with music came dance. I loved to dance and so did my family. My sister loved to dance too. She always did it secretly so no one could judge her skills. The first time I saw her dance she was probably seventeen and I was sixteen, and I was like, wow girl you *can* dance! And we had that stress as a community: Can you dance? That was a question people expected you to say yes to. It was an entry ticket to belonging to the lion's share of any group of people near me. I'll talk more about dance a little later when I suggest that dance is Buddha Dharma.

Some songs and dances later proved to be pure sexual coos delivering directions directly to the subconscious, especially influencing misuse of sex and sexuality. A lot of the songs, some of which I listen to today when I feel like I need to reconnect to my culture and reflect, created insane beliefs in my consciousness. For example, somebody, the songs promised, of the right gender energy was going to woo me into happiness, and dance was going to free me from all suffering by lying within the arms of another. Or the songs promised to transfer me right on into heaven and gave me a recipe for finding that perfect partner and overcoming racial and gender tensions within the Black community. These cultural tools served to shape mine and others existences for decades, and really kept me going in circles since I believed in the promises given in these songs and let myself delve into dance. We could leave our nine-to-five up on the shelf and just enjoy ourselves, like Michael Jackson told us to. Or just close the door baby, said Teddy Pendergrass, or dance our way out of our constrictions, said ConFunkShun, and it would all be okay. That was total delusion and distraction to ignore and diminish the feelings of being alone and separate, and the confused and fear-based thoughts of not knowing what life was about, why there was racism, incest, alcoholism and addiction, war, deformed babies, poverty—suffering in general.

1. Cultural Norms and Conditions

Let's Eat!

Music and dance weren't the only cultural hooks. Food. Now that's a big one. At the time I was growing up, people were using Crisco and eating breaded then fried meats and fish, and casseroles, lots of homemade cakes and pies, corn bread, pork and potatoes. White bread and mayonnaise, bologna, American cheese, donuts, stuff like that. Yes, I was a fat child. It took a few decades for me to learn how to eat so that I wouldn't die of Type 2 diabetes! And what I wore depended on my weight. A lot of classmates were wearing what was in style each year. No, not me. My clothes had to be specially made to fit. And trust me, they weren't stylish at all. And my father made us wear orthopedic shoes to school so our feet wouldn't be misshapen. You get the picture?

Those norms of food had everything to do with how poor American Blacks were marginalized and had to eat substandard foods due to the history of antiblack racism and lack of food equities in the poor neighborhoods and whatnot. Some of us associate foods with stereotypes and bigotry. Even today, a few American Black people I interact with won't eat Mexican, Indian, or other ethnic foods since they think they're better than people with such lineage, or they associate such foods with lack. My uncle, an American Black man, wouldn't drink coffee; he swore coffee makes you black.

Clearly, eating can turn into addiction. People eat to change their feelings, they overeat, or don't eat enough if they're anorexic and bulimic by choice or don't have money to spend on food. The relationship between nutrition and food has been lost for some people. A lot of us have no idea how food comes to us these days or that food in packages isn't always "food." In fact, I didn't learn about nutritious food until I went to college. And as I said, I was overweight. As a young teen, during junior high I was anorexic and continued that addiction through my young adult life. I always thought I was fat. I felt this way even though I had maintained a healthy weight, all the way through to the MM diagnosis, when I dropped weight so fast it wasn't funny. At that point I wished I had had a different perspective.

For many, eating is done in secret when anxiety, fear, or boredom gets really great. Eating while doing something else, like reading or driving or reading the mobile phone, also contributes to food addictions. When eating, no other activity should be going on. Just focus on eating, and how the wholesome food has been arranged, where it came from. Do you know how many labors came together to make wholesome food available for you?

In an early childhood neighborhood of mine, there were gangs and thugs who would terrorize the streets. With no car, my mother, me, and my sisters walked to the grocery store trying to avoid the gang members. My mother bought expired foods, low-quality produce, tainted meats, with food stamps. We carried bags back to the apartment hoping that we wouldn't get jacked on the way there. As important as food is to individual and collective well-being, these retail practices still exist today. Many people who have enough nutritious wholesome food to eat are deluded into thinking that we are better than people in lower class neighborhoods who are suffering these kinds of food deserts. This is thinking that keeps us believing we are separate from each other.

Food is a great healer or a great disease purveyor. Many of the diseases that become "natural causes" of death, including cancer, could be held at bay if foods were eaten for nutrition and health, rather than as a drug or an escape. Of course, the occasional treat is probably okay. Leaving aside highly processed foods, drinks, alcohol, high-fat meats, and sugary goods should take priority. While it is true that anyone no matter what could get cancer or other diseases regardless of the foods they chose, the data show that having a diet of whole grains, nuts, omega fishes, lean meat and poultry, low-fat dairy, vegetables, and legumes generally is more beneficial to sustain life (Donaldson, 2004), and that, in turn, allows you the ability to help more people!

You Wearing What? You Driving That?

Clothes are definitely what make you who you are in a lot of American Black communities. I don't even feel like I need to say anything more about this as it seems evident. I can't assume that though, so I will. Churches. School. Workplaces. Your outfit arrives before you can say a word. People talk about your clothes well after they're out of sight. Clothes are ways to develop and produce a self, an identity. The clothes are hanging on the ego all day and night. And the same can be said about vehicles. The vehicle you drive is your signature. I'm not saying having nice things is wrong or right. I'm saying look at why you want them, what you want them for, and how they make you feel. When you have them, then what? When you don't have them, what then? They're just signifiers. In themselves clothes mean nothing. They're just signifying an idea. So we also know that the advertisers and the fashion industry want us to believe something else. If you have had children you know the drill. If you're a clothes horse, you know the drill. A good deal of the clothes we buy wind up in a landfill here, or overseas in poor countries. They say that it amounts to 81.5 pounds per person per year. That's after the puny 15 percent that is kept and sold through recycling at your local donation store. And get this: 2,150 textile pieces are discarded per second across the United States (Ingini, 2023). So ask yourself if you or your children need those clothes. Also consider that we are all connected and this is a perfect lens through which this can be seen. Nearly half of the garments are in poor condition when they're dumped into developing countries, like Ghana and Chile, as a secondhand marketplace, or in the oceans. Loads of discarded clothing can't be sold in a secondhand market for the reason that they're in bad shape (Besser, 2021). It's definitely a crisis. So while clothes and vehicles used to be status symbols for American Blacks when owning real property wasn't available to us and before the fast discardable clothing industry developed, thinking carefully about what is needed is a critical step. When we throw something away, it sits on the earth somewhere. Clothes are no different, neither are vehicles. They have to go somewhere too when they're broken down and unusable. Like I've said, I don't mean we have to look awful or drive vehicles barely making it. I'm suggesting we pay attention to our purchases from an ego point of view. I'm moving on now, since I think I made a point here about how we can break our attachment to clothing, and vehicles, and look at how it's driven from ego.

Gender and Domestic Violence

So a lot of greed and hate through delusion is inflicted by American Blacks and other people of color on each other. Car thefts, burglaries, killings, incest, domestic violence, rape, male dominance, religious and other scams, and all manner of unwholesome actions are the norm, every day. These kinds of attacks have been going on for generations of American Black people. These abuses were overlain or underpinned by the dome of centuries of being abused by others too. In addition to the cultural perspectives I talked about earlier, the shaping of our consciousnesses was made in our minds individually and collectively, geographically, and globally. These shapes form excuses for and approval of discrimination within our communities as well as without. These are also the bases for building egos. That is to say, believing internally, *"I'm better than you."*

In learning an identity, people internalize messages about how to behave and think depending on their gender, whether they align with their birth sex organs or not. All of us are assumed to be male or female from the outset, and nowadays some people explore alternatives during the formative years or over time. I don't want to generalize anything; I'm just saying that whatever gender identity is adapted, it contributes to the egoic self and colors responses and reactions to internal and external perception of objects of the mind. In my case as a female-identified person, I was very strongly attached to nail polish, hairdos, dresses, makeup, frilly things, and high-heeled shoes. I wanted to be the one courted and cherished, asked out on dates, and have my doors opened for me. You get the point. As I became more attentive to my ego, when this wasn't happening for me, I got upset. Why? After I posed an inquiry into why I got angry, I found that my ego said I was *supposed* to receive all the accoutrements of the feminine. Then I discovered that those were just ideas and projections placed into my ego consciousness by outside sources. Now I can still want those acknowledgments, without being attached to them if I don't get them. More to the point, I have dropped many of them with the view that they don't support seeing life as it is, so when I do feel like "I want" I can take a second and pose additional inquiry. How does this help others? Who does it hurt? Is it a right action? A beneficial action? An identity action?[1]

Objects of mind are very numerous, and they can be tangible things or intangible ideas, thoughts, feelings, or projections into the future, beliefs about the past, and like I mentioned they're being created from the time we're born. Women are supposed to be soft and dainty, wait for the man to make decisions, raise the children, be motherly and never get angry. Men are supposed to be strong, powerful, bringing protection, discipline, and financial stability to the family and are allowed—expected—to get angry. Children are supposed to obey and worship their parents. These are basic sorts of rules of a family that are portrayed in many cultural spaces around the world. Movies and television, politicians, as well as talk-show hosts and podcasters, teach and revere this kind of family. These gender roles are supported by religious doctrines in many cases. We can imagine that often these portrayals are abjectly different from the actual home, totally unrealistic.

Recently I was talking with someone who has a master's degree in social work, and they were saying that many domestic violence homes are that way, being that beatings are cultural expressions of love. They said this is why people don't leave and more often than not, when they do leave eventually return to the abuser. Next, I asked him if it was so much about love, why do some people wind up dead? He just shrugged at that and couldn't answer. Being beaten or having any kind of physical abuse, whether from throwing things, breaking belongings, and so on, isn't love as I understand it. Other types of abuse are more subtle, like name calling, gaslighting, and ghosting or manipulations and bullying. Neither I nor this book provides counseling for domestic violence and abuse. Rather, the point is meant to bring light to the fact that it's ego driven. Anger is from ego, not getting what is wanted; that is to say, it brings harm whereas it demands something from someone to satisfy anger. Or to get the upper hand. Dominate. Domestic abuse doesn't leave any income level out, either. It happens all over, in all neighborhoods.

As women are socialized to be dainty, and men are supposed to be strong, American Black men are often devalued in American society, and not able to achieve the strong male persona. We see this through many depictions in newscasts, employment and education statistics, and addiction rates. Regardless, there are many successful Black men that don't get any countenance from anyone on any scales. Many men throughout all strata of American Black society look for and expect to receive the respect they need from the family. And women seek equality and respect from their male counterparts, as they themselves have to deal with racial discrimination and thoughts and feelings of powerlessness too. All of this involves ego. If we can drop the ego, we can heal.

At the same time, the racial structures that have been imbedded in the wider superstructure have given rise to our belief in some of the messages, one that is particularly damaging: that people of African heritage can't be trusted, aren't intellectual, can't do math or science, idiotic labels like that, and these are swishing around within American Black people's heads whether we acknowledge them or not. Everyone who is born in the United States eventually comes to reality with these centuries of beliefs ingrained in collective unconsciousness. And we see or hear with a clouded view of who we are and who the other person is, believing we are separate from each other.

We all desire and need love from people. That's just human. Love in the right way. Healthy love. Love that doesn't arise from egoistic demands. It arises from wanting to help others without reward or acknowledgment. The way to get love we want is to give love.

As humans, we're driven by a self and ego that, for an appreciable number of us, we are totally unaware of, and we try to grasp and hold onto an impermanent life, which is called emptiness.[2] Nothing is permanent as much as we deny it to be so, and this informs the ego and self, too. This drive has to be questioned and examined by each person in order to see the belief in the self and the manifesting of ego. In terms of overcoming it, what we have to do is to change how we see, look at our responses, to take the time to wait, let go of just going along with the program. Ask why do I want this or why do I believe this, and where do these desires and points of view originate? Why am I attached to them? Do they really define who I am? This is a way of inquiry that allows us to see that our reactions and responses can be very much out of our control. The way forward is to see through the ego and the automatic nature of a conditioned belief in a self that has been created by beliefs that are destructive in the long run.

Addictions

I talked about food addictions earlier. Thousands of people are addicted to something to some degree, even if it's addiction to recovery or meditation. Those who get into recovery may switch to attending too many meetings for their habit of choice. That's okay for a while, as are all temporary strategies to overcome destructive addictive behavior.

Addiction comes in internal and external forms and can, in unchecked cases, cause long-term financial, emotional, mental, and physical harm. If we meditate all day to the exclusion of our responsibilities there are consequences, just like if we drink or use drugs, etc., in the same way. Addiction is a source of relief that temporarily makes us feel good, or is used to provide some escape from suffering, gone haywire. You can be addicted to a person, such as someone who abuses you constantly and won't stop, and abuse comes in verbal, mental, emotional, and physical forms. You think it's the other person with the problem; in all honesty really, it's both of you. If only they would change, you keep thinking. Honestly, you need to change too. These people are at home and at work, at places of worship, at school, basically anywhere we interact with others. A real example of addiction to people is codependency such as in domestic violence and incestuous situations, where parents try to control their children with abuse. Or consider work-related oppressions with self-centered coworkers, owners, and managers, places where children are molested such as churches and organized groups.

Of course, there are substance addictions, all drugs, alcohol, and tobacco, foods, and drinks. Many of the processed foods are produced to get you hooked, and they can cause mental and physical damage to you for a long time. The thing is that these are more acute in neighborhoods of low-income people of color, and access to resources is somewhat less than in more affluent areas. And let's not leave out addictions to buying stuff, gambling, compulsive lying, pornography, the euphoria of new sexual relationships with a new one every year or so after the thrill is gone, social media where nothing is real, keeping the realities away to change the focus for a bit of time. Each incident of addiction engagement pushes you into a worse position.

If you change a response or a behavior, often the situation will change, now that the habit energy pattern is broken. From a cultural perspective we think we're stuck and have no way out, since maybe this is the way it's been done in the family forever and a day. And it's not to be spoken of. We create habits of mind in order to cope with the underlying fears, shame, and feelings of being unloved or inadequate, stupid, helpless, separate, and resolve to just give up and give in. Or if we do try to change ourselves, we try to do it alone, saying we don't need any help. Or we make up excuses about how we can't do it, shielded by thoughts like we don't have the money, time, transportation, support, or how we are treated differently, the system is broken, and so on. These excuses are all manifestations of ego, self-delusions, the mind keeping you from being your best self, your true self.

Education

This isn't in any way equitable or equal and it never has been in the history of American Blacks in the United States. Even today, places of education are rife with cultural messages that place people on particular paths, and a place where we learn about bootstraps and hard work. Educational institutions, even homeschooling, are hierarchical, and scores of them are exclusionary or discriminating in some way (in Chapter 5 I'll talk about an American Black woman-led boarding school that only accepted wealthy American Blacks). Each of them can be damaging by leaving out information or emphasizing other information such as the importance of studying certain subjects or the rigor of the curriculum. Overworked parents, who have no support, or who are unable to meet the demands of educating their children, rely on what's available to them. And every child deserves and needs a fair and substantial education, which includes studies that provide access to be able to work in technology, science, political discourse, to understand critical thinking, to assess and evaluate situations, arts, and know humanities and social sciences to a degree that is equivalent to the highest standards when they graduate from high school. Not everyone wants this and in many cases they don't want it, feeling they have already been beaten down and believing they can't achieve any of this, or that it's unnecessary, as a result of the cultural orientation they are in. True, some have the ability and the means. Instead, for whatever reason, they turn away from it. Let me not forget to say that if admitted to university or college, not an American Black college, it's often very difficult to complete. Classes are extremely unrelenting; sources of support are there, but availing them is difficult normally, resulting from not knowing how to access them, or from being ashamed, thinking we don't need them.

All this being true, education is the key to knowing how to evaluate yourself, and your ego, to be able to sincerely determine if you're being led astray and using your human mind appropriately. If you do not know how to think, there is difficulty in finding your way out of consequences that arise from causes and conditions and thinking critically about your actions and intentions to ascertain their short- and long-term impact on you and those you affect. By having appropriate knowledge, coupled with right action, intuition, and wisdom, it's likely that causes and conditions perpetuated by egos can be mitigated, preventing the centuries of oppression through antiblack racism from continuing to be repeated. It starts with one person, and it affects and spreads to those around them at home, at the park, at the store. At work.

Work

For me, getting a job was a ticket out of my childhood home. It was crazy broke there it seemed, with my mother then being the only one making any money after my father's death. She didn't ever have enough for three children.

Part One

American culture overall is mesmerized by money and getting a lot of it and thrives on the consumption machine driven by people working and buying. You can't do anything here without money. Everything is monetized, all the way down to buying air for your flat tire at the gas station. Stuff that's for sale, whether it's an Internet connection or an interest rate, is categorized into markets and market segments. Market segments are comprised of people's buying power based on economics on the one hand, and preferences on the other. Not everyone's Internet connection speed or bandwidth is created equal, and we all don't get the same interest rates on anything. Big corporations and money markets usually get all the profits.

Enter the verb "to work." If America is obsessed with buying, its obsession is met by work. People who get the best Internet speeds and interest rates are people with high credit ratings, and these are people who generally have the best work arrangements, make a high salary, have a certain kind of education, and who are male identified. These people are working in a system that is connected to retirement, banking, credit markets, health care, and the network of processes that are established based on the cultural norms. These norms are not just American based, creeping in, accepted as a normative way of being in Western countries. At home, school, and at religious establishments, in media programing, social media, and from stories about your family's fortune hidden in a mattress, we are socialized to get a job, to be self-sufficient, to help the family, to get up and get off the parent's pocketbook. Be independent. Of course, not all families are like this; some are so wealthy, or some have made successes, so that these conversations and programming do not occur. And some are generationally uninclined to get a job that requires a Social Security number or a bank account. They subsist or find parity of income through engaging in purveying not so legal goods and services. Here I'm focused on the messages for those of us who work ourselves to death with no rest, regardless of what they do.

Go to college, go to the military, or get a job. This is the mantra for many households in the country in order to feed the consumption machine. First of all, if you go to the military *without* a college degree you'll be put at the lowest rank. They say go to college. The statement should be *graduate* from a *good* college. That's when you can maybe qualify for a decent job. At the same time, unless you're a successful entrepreneur, the entry into the work world with good credentials still requires continuous hard work. And some people choose professions that are not well suited to their personalities and tendencies. This is what's called selecting a profession in order to be wealthy, rather than engaging "right livelihood." Right livelihood is working in a field that doesn't cause harm to you or others, and these roles might not pay very well even though they may require extensive education. Roles in these veins often ask that the roar of the consumption machine be toned down and actually turned off.

Unfortunately, it doesn't often get toned down or turned off. People turn to selling illegally with the sole goal of making money outside the system, often in response to the causes and conditions they live in that keep them out of the system, even if they choose right livelihood. Of course, there are those in the system who also turn to illegal transactions in cash or though scams and so on. My point is that there are many people who are left out of the ability to work and earn a right living, coming from the cultural causes and conditions. In many couple-based African American households, the female energy is granted the privilege of getting a job while the male energy doesn't get a break at all. And this has been an imposed way of life for centuries through antiblack racism. That conditioning feeds the feelings of inadequacy for both people, as they watch the stories of families in shows and movies that do not reflect their circumstance, or they watch shows that perpetuate American Black people being portrayed in negative situations.

In neighborhoods around the United States, American Black men are unemployed and are seen standing outside, hanging around. What is your response when you see this anywhere? For people within American Black cultural strata, those who have been able to find a fulltime job maybe think, why don't they get a job or at least stop standing on the corner? All sorts of assumptions based in antiblack racism dictate these thoughts. And as is the case in everything we see, we only see a tiny fraction of the whole situation. When I think perhaps that they shouldn't be standing around like that, what judgments am I making? Where is my ego in my thought base? Is it trying to make sure the signals of drug dealing don't manifest so I don't suffer? In other words, am I putting myself above them and thinking only of what consequences could come to *me* if the men are habitually hanging out? Does it mean I can't go outside safely? I'm not saying these aren't relevant concerns in a given situation. I'm saying that the ego is running the show and it has to be moved off center stage. Zen Buddhist practice helps with this.

I have to say I worked myself to a point of fatigue until I was forced to retire through bodily collapse and a diagnosis of terminal blood cancer. My working career began at age fourteen and continued nonstop until age sixty-two. When I retired, I realized all the striving, in view of the fact that I wasn't in a Right Livelihood environment, and my ego talked me into taking on too much, being ambitious even though I had what I believed were good motives, driven by an emotion that I recognize now as not feeling loved, and I collapsed. It was also at that time that I realized the toll antiblack racism had on me. There were positions I didn't get, acknowledgments not offered, money not forthcoming on the slide from antiblack racism on the one hand from whites. On the other hand was equally disappointing treatment from people of color who were in the position to do these things, instead relied on bigotry to make their decisions. It seemed like my efforts were in vain. Competitive behaviors and interracial and intraracial antiblack discrimination just beat me to a pulp. Still, examining my ego and belief in a separate self has helped me to find some joy and ease, as well as understanding the emptiness of all ambition-based striving and blaming. It has made me attentive to the human conditioned reality and the ultimate reality of Buddha Mind as we live within the two.

Loyalties

The food, music, dance, religion—all the cultural perspectives—create social loyalties. You eat what your family serves at gatherings to keep the peace, or you keep going to the church even though you have long ago stopped finding any solace there, if you ever did. You don't tell your close friends the truth about their addictions with love in your heart, you don't want to hurt them or lose them. You see that buying stuff doesn't actually make you feel better for very long, or that you've chosen a job that keeps you sad and depressed, believing you need the money. Search deeply and you'll find that the ego is in control. You dare not say no thanks to that butter poundcake as you don't want to hurt feelings, I mean after all they made it just for you, and plus, you're the golden child so you can't disappoint. Or you dare not stop going to the church. What will people think? You get a new car or move to a new spot, or get in or out of a relationship situation. What does all that do besides make you feel empty and needing more? This is suffering. How can we see clearly in such a way as to actualize a new view, a clearer understanding of reality, a way that unhooks cultural norms from ego self-centered drives, and more importantly addresses antiblack racism from inside of being black with appropriate responses? The interesting realization is that the loyalty is to an object or an idea that enforces a view of being separate from other people, as well as enforcing the constructed self, which is attached to your ego. Let's do this: Select an object such as a pair of shoes or a movie or an athletic event, or an idea of a neighborhood, an *alma mater* or a club, including a gang, you belong to. The shoes could be Timberlands, the movie could be *Black Panther*, and the athletic event could be a competition between top-ranked teams. If you don't have loyalty to a team, that's fine, you could use a sorority or a fraternity. Someone steps on your shoe and gets them dirty with a smudge that can't be cleaned. What happens? Why? Is it that the shoes represent your loyalty to a self you have constructed? Or someone says the movie was super stupid and had no bearing in changing people's perceptions. What happens? Why? You are committed to the idea that how Black people have been cast in the last three-quarter century is wrong and white people should change. Your team loses and you're ready to fight. Why? You are loyal to it as it represents a part of you from the past or a place where you fit in and you want to maintain that since it gives an identity to you, and your ego revels in being accepted. Loyalty means you won't leave, regardless of the price you pay. What price are you paying to remain loyal to unhealthy objects and ideas that only maintain the ego and keep you from opening your mind a hair's breadth?

We pay the price to avoid being labeled fools, chumps, suckers, called Uncle Tom, or any manner of names American Blacks hurl at each other for bucking the American Black system, which means we are going to the white system, that insults the ego. There is a middle place to land, not only the white or black sides.

I heard a Dharma talk not too long ago from a Dharma teacher recounting a story about her giving money to a homeless couple. At first, her ego felt good about it, although she had some trepidation when she pulled out her wallet on the city street corner. When she crossed the street after giving up $15 so the couple could get a place to sleep for the night, a woman standing nearby promptly told her that those people had been standing on the corner all day collecting $15 from many people so they can do drugs. She told us what her ego said after she heard that: *you a fool, you crazy, you just a chump, you shouldn't give homeless people money, why don't you go back and get the money*? Then after a few minutes of examining her egoic thinking, self-obsessed to the max, she said, overtaken by greed, hate, and delusion, she remembered that she doesn't have to be loyal to the idea of "not being taken" by "someone trying to get over." The obligation is to only recognize delusion and speak to it. What does it matter if they do drugs with the money? It was a gift and that doesn't change with a remark. How many times have I given a gift only to find that it wasn't used the way it I thought it should have been used or that I gave it not knowing the full picture, that they would pawn it or barter it? Regift it? It's still a gift. I'll talk about generosity within the context of *the Wisdom Paramitas* later in the book. For now, the questions are, can you walk around with a smudge on your shoe? Or can you see the shoes for what they are rather than attach to them as they represent your constructed identity? Can you abstain from watching All Black movies and television? Or can you interpret the movies and shows differently? Can your team lose and you not be angry? Can you vigorously root for the other team without fear? Loyalty runs deep, feeding the ego and the self in ways that keep us separate, stuck in beliefs that may not be skillful.

Religion

Lots of religions make promises, telling us that our best chance of happiness is in the next life or after death. If we do good, we'll get good. If we pray right, we'll get right. If we give, we'll get. If we obey God, we'll overcome. Religion has been the go to place for American Blacks for centuries. Religions keep the self in the forefront. If we keep the commandments we'll be seen as holy. It's about what we're getting, about our self, and that's in turn attached to egos. Some have been turning away or leaving the church—breaking their loyalties. And some aren't. What I want to bring to your consciousness is an idea that the church can perpetuate antiblack racism in the minds of American Blacks. Be that as it may, the conversation about Zen Buddhism geared toward people like me is absconded on the one hand, seeing that Zen Buddhist centers are generally predominately white, and a white person can't address antiblack racism directly with American Blacks, and on the other, American Black people are not likely to embrace any Buddhism practice, particularly since they don't know of it. In my case, I hadn't encountered Buddhism until I was well into midlife and visited Tassajara Mountain Zen Center for a guest stay. Nonetheless, if some do encounter Buddhism, there is fear of engaging with it. Historical beliefs and Christian teachings usually disallow trying other religious practices. Assuming though we overcome that barrier, some may perceive antiblack racism at Buddhist centers. Much of that is due to the way a practice container is set up, by not making eye contact, being quiet, working collectively, wearing specific clothing, or by having food that's vegetarian and based on Asian cuisine. It's true that there are some folks who don't know what to do when they encounter a person of color. So they may say something unwholesome. Plenty of places nowadays have strong affinities for diversity, equity, and inclusion, and they make deep efforts to welcome everyone, all cultures, all genders, all ages, religious backgrounds, sexual identities, and so forth. I haven't experienced any sense of racism from people who lead Buddhist centers and monasteries.

Zen Buddhism

Zen Buddhism doesn't promise anything. No heaven, no hell. No bliss. No escape from racism. Zen Buddhism wants us to find the Middle Way. I'll concede that trying to find the middle ground between historical antiblack racism and experiential racism of today and the way these manifest as causes and conditions are difficult to grapple with. Zen Buddhism is also very concerned with the questions surrounding life and death, and what we're doing here, questions that are never the direct ones underpinning antiblack racism.

Buddhism has different schools, you know? Each of them addresses the issue of what happens after death using the idea of karma, or, stated differently, causes and conditions. That is to say that birth and death, or suffering, make up a cycle and one can leave the cycle of suffering with practice realization. This is the way that can be used to transform the ego from self-oriented to realizing a connection to all beings and things orientation. When you hurt, everyone hurts, for example. The concept of an "original face," before any historical and cultural labels were placed on you, tells us we are all sharing a value embedded in humanity, which is there for illuminating. We only have to become attuned to the fact of it. Within the original face there is no difference, no discrimination, no separation between us and other people on the planet. Getting attuned to it allows us to exhibit compassion and loving kindness, to learn how to return an appropriate response in any situation.

Within the Zen Buddhist community all are welcome and there is no requirement to leave any religious affiliation. The emphasis is on sitting meditation, or Zazen, learning to identify the self that propels us into unskillful situations, and to be able to slow it down until we can actually stop it from controlling our every thought, habit-energy reactions, business, and putting ourselves down all day every day from fear. We learn instead to see both our perfections and imperfections without judgment, tempered with the understanding that it's the ego, formed by our cultural conditioning, that drives us. When we are able to see this, a new world opens before us. Whether you have had a deep experience with organized religion, none at all, or don't believe in a monotheistic deity, Zen Buddhism welcomes you just as you are. Yes, I know, you've likely heard that before. The good news is you'll be exploring topics and given freedom to make your own evaluation, to go with what you've learned or to drop it any time. There's no proselytizing and in fact there is a lot of "I don't know" that goes on about questions, so we can be comfortable with not having the answers to everything. At the same time, our sort of way we work in the physical world is to ask, How can I help? rather than, What am I going to get? We do know that everything that is experienced or produced on earth is impermanent, and will decay or change over time, even if the time period is undetectable to our human experience.

Everyone suffers in this life no matter how it appears to you. And there is a way out of suffering. The Buddha's *Four Noble Truths* tell us exactly this:

1. There is suffering.
2. There is a cause of suffering.
3. There is freedom from suffering.
4. There is a Path of Liberation from Suffering.

These truths are a way of dropping ego, and in turn, antiblack racism for American Blacks.

Opening to Zen Buddhism can soothe the sores of antiblack racism that American Blacks and other people of color try to cover up and deny or ignore. Taking up the practice, we learn the role of the mind, we are not separate from others, intentions are the roots of causes and conditions, everyone is suffering, and our egos drive us to act. It is important to offer this medicine to us, and at the same time, have privileged classes continue to be self-reflective and accountable to ending antiblack racism.

Part One

During COVID many displays of antiblack racism were shown on screens around the world, to some viewers' "surprise." At the same time, giving time to those displays, many white people engaged in studying their roles in keeping antiblack racism and its negative impacts alive and how they could change their beliefs and behaviors. I want to acknowledge and own how American Black people stabilize antiblack racism also unknown to them and give some ideas of how our beliefs and behaviors may change by practicing Zen Buddhism.

As a point of reference, bigotry heavily exists within nondominant groups; it's called bigotry knowing that nondominant groups don't have controls of networks to enforce racism. Bigotry hurts not only individuals, but also generations of families, and societies. That in turn creates entanglements that both place people of color at disadvantage relative to dominate culture and create bigotry intra- and interculturally. As a small example, consider bringing a potential spouse of the "wrong" race, or religion, or ethnicity, or age, or sexual preference, or economic and social status, to a family gathering. Some families go nuts over this and it causes escalated hate and separation issues.

Zazen meditation, along with living within *Wisdom Practices*, embodying Buddhist vows and adhering to related precepts, creates space to reduce suffering and separation. In turn, these bring clarity and the reduction of or at least awareness of reactions, reactions stemming from cultural habit energy. The precepts, vows, and wisdom practices are there to help to cultivate the soil where individual and generational karma can be dealt with, to see the self and the belief in separateness clearly as they are. This allows the ability to come from the place of reducing harm, to helping others to develop different responses, and therefore different causes and conditions can prevail. The ripple effect starts in relationships, with family, friends, and others, bringing the way out of bigotry to the larger society.

The change in perspective gives empowerment and agency, which is actually what one seeks in victimhood. First, each of us—racists and bigots to some degree I'd suggest, as we see differences—needs to do our own work, personally and then collectively. After that work is done, then we can create spaces for safe dialog, after we have let go of holding tightly to ego. Next, there's the skillful way of understanding the humanity within the group, then between the groups, then more globally.

2

Ways of Living for American Blacks

Apply Zen Buddhist Practices

See that you see differently than before Awakening
This Radiant Light is Everywhere in All things at All times
—Tanahashi, 2013, p. 415

In Chapter 1, I talked about cultural conditioning and how it can control who we are. In this chapter I'm going to go over some main points of Zen Buddhism. They include how dualistic thinking and self-centeredness can lead to unclear seeing. Then I'll talk about causes and conditions: One of the main ways that we get stuck in a thinking pattern is through following the well-trod path of attaining, fame, gain, and going after what we think we should be driving for. Next I'll talk about the notions of greed, hate and anger, and delusion. After that, the next part of this chapter goes into what's known as emptiness and impermanence, understanding of which helps move us away from self-centeredness. I'll spend some time here, then go on to review the Buddha's awakening, the *Wisdom Paramitas*, and living by vow. Then, I'll get to Zazen, which is the meditation practice Zen Buddhism.

Dualistic Thinking

Right, wrong, good, bad, black, white, rich, poor. Everything in this world is conditioned within duality. She's ugly, he's a player.

They're lazy. Now the family across the way, each of the folks has two jobs and that's good. With dualistic thinking there's often judgment and a value proposition. We live in this world, and to make some order out of it, you have to be able to think and operate within dualities. You wouldn't be able to drive to a destination or make a cake or construct a building if there weren't any. Nor would you be able to determine the quality of anything if we didn't have the ability to use comparisons to assess situations and things.

The main issue with duality, though, is thinking that you're the center of the universe, where everything revolves around you, the home of the ego itself. That everything you see is in relation to you at the center, with everything else as objects. Your clothes, the food you eat, the place you live, your friends and family, people you work with, the gifts you give, these are all seen as objects. And objectifying means you see these as separate from yourself, completely outside of yourself, just something to be used for personal gain or satisfaction. In countless cases when we aren't attentive in the Zen Buddhist sense of the word, we have no idea that we are so self-absorbed.

Self-Centered and Self-Disliked

Being self-centered, self-disliking, and self-absorbed, self-obsessed, and self-oriented isn't something new. We are all that way at some point before encountering and practicing Zen Buddhism. Even after a steady practice we can still be this way. It's not something to dislike—it's something to notice. Everything revolves around us, what we want or don't want, the goals we are encouraged to set, designing the life we want. Or, we are focused on self by giving up and giving in, resolving it's no use, no one cares, why bother. On both sides of this coin, we don't like ourselves remembering or knowing of the ways we behave on occasions, or the way we react or feel. Often we don't know what else to do. You want to be different, feel different, maybe stop being so anxious, scared, or cowardly. Or we want to stop being so aggressive and angry, for example. Greedy at whatever we're doing. We want to have good relationships and treat people with kindness, including treating ourselves with kindness. We don't know how. Our reactions are automatic, at least it seems, plain old habitually doing what has always been done. Then we feel bad about them and go off and do some addictive thing, like buying something or eating something or whatever to help us feel better. Instead, we feel worse. It's a hamster wheel, right? And then, we have justifications for how we feel bad—it's not my fault, they're cheating me, she's always been like that, or I don't trust them—so we can't dig out of the hole of the habit energy of blame and shame.

And it's not our fault on a grander level. We've been taught to attach to achievement, competition, and outwardly focus on what will make us happy. It's formulaic, and it's typically based in the American cultural delusion backed by consumption, capitalism, the set of family values I talked about in the prior chapter, and on a Christian-based ethos, from both the Old and New Testaments. We haven't been encouraged at all to look at the notion of causes and conditions of happiness. Those notions, instead, are based on making an appropriate response, not automatically reacting to a situation, as well as thinking about other people, not just us, thinking of how we impact those around us.

Causes and Conditions

We were born into this world, landing smacked into patriarchy, oppression, racism. These conditions arose from beginningless time, greed, hate, and delusion from a collective past. The situation was set when we were born. And the causes? No one knows exactly. This questioning of why, wanting to know what happened, is a nice foray.

What is relevant is looking at causes and conditions you can impact yourself. Instead of living as a deluded person, we can live by vow, where we consciously look to help others, to have compassion, to let go of self. Grasping for happiness, allowing anger to guide our reactions, and not seeing the actual reality occurring in front of us keep us blind to the fact that we can eliminate our suffering. Happiness comes to us and remains with us, when we don't place it as a center goal, when we aren't adhering tightly to specific wants and desires on our terms, our preferences, rather that we live from vow and a constancy of practice. It's that we know we are not separate from each other and that trying to help one another can reduce our sense of suffering and our reactions to it.

Getting Out of Grasping

Sands passing through fingers, memories, dreams, hopes, wants, and expectations: Does anyone actually get what they want, or remember the past as it was? It's a dream that we can't wake up from. We don't see it clearly, no matter how hard we try or feel that our memory is correct. For the future dream, in the Western world, many experts tell us that we have to plan our goals, chart our courses, and be self-reliant. Then there are individuals and organizations that cry out, exalt, and promise fantastic results, if only we attract what we want, pray earnestly for particulars in detail: a spouse with certain qualities, a house, a career, family, children, cars—the list is endless; being part of the human condition, desire lives unbridled and unidentified in many of us, although the attainment of each goal only leads to desire for more with further unhappiness and delusion resulting, inasmuch as nothing is permanent.

The truth of the matter is that fulfilling those desires is never enough to answer the need we have for love and acceptance, and this is the beginning of accepting personal powerlessness as expounded in the Twelve Step programs. People try to behave in ways that will somehow fill the central hole, or the need for community, wholesome community, by taking in unwholesome people, places, and things to the detriment of self and others. It's a feeling of separateness. A cry of desperation for help we don't know how to ask for.

Causes are the outcomes from actions, and being attached to wanting or desire. I desire something, thinking it's going to make me better or relieve my suffering. I go after it. I get it. It isn't what I expected. I'm hurt. I try to get out of that pain. So I desire something else, grasping again. Thinking that will help me feel happy. And the cycle continues.

Greed, Hate and Anger, and Delusion

Wanting more can be characterized as greed. It can be trying to make the unspoken knowledge or feelings of impermanence go away. It can be more than that even, as in wanting what you want and wanting it now, without considering the impact on others. Greed can be taking out of the earth more than is useful or skillful. In short, greed is the human condition we have been dealt, to deal with shoring up assurances against running out before we die. Running out of material goods, love, friendship, safety, not belonging to the correct group. Not knowing what happens at death, or why we have to face life and death. You name it, greed can run our lives directly into the ground. The online search for the meaning of greed returned "intense and selfish desire for something, especially wealth, power, or food." Covetousness, craving, desire, impatience are some other words that describe greed. Wikipedia authors talk about greed being insatiable desire for those mentioned just now, as well and also for social status or value. Further, greed creates conflict between personal and social goals, or, stated in Zen Buddhist terms, it creates a separation between self and others. Oftentimes, greed leads to lying, stealing, self-aggrandizement. It can also lead to hate and anger.

I want to take these two terms separately.

What is hate? We know what that is from antiblack racism and other racist practices, misogyny, patriarchy, stances against different sexual orientations, and so on. These kinds of hate stem from revulsive feelings, and from beliefs that one thinks they're better than another. Hate is a feeling of intense or passionate dislike for someone or group, set of ideas, or a belief system. You can simultaneously hate a group or a person from a group, while at the same time smiling at them. Hate can be both macro and micro in scope, and at the same time selective. For example, you may have a person in your family that you accept from a group outside of your ethnic, sexual, or religious practice. Simultaneously, though, you at the same time hate the representative group.

How is hate different from anger? Anger brings annoyance, displeasure, frustration, or irrigation. You can be angry that someone got

---

a promotion or a better deal than you. Or you can be angry that your son or daughter married a person you didn't approve of. Generally, fear is behind anger: You're not getting what you want or you may lose what you have. You're scared, you're worried or have sadness about an outcome. Anger can be subsumed in hate. It comes especially when hate is rooted in racism, a sense of privilege, patriarchy, etc. Anger is temporary and can often be addressed. Viscerally, hate underlies, provokes, and establishes the creation of personal, financial, legal, and social power over other groups. It takes away one's humanity, completely, with a learned idea of being better than those in the targeted group.

What about delusion? Yes, hate is a delusion carried out, enacted, and creating harm. Unfortunately we all live in delusion of some form or other. We think reality is one way; in actuality, really, it's hard to tell what reality is usually. Even with evidence to the contrary, we believe the delusions we cloud ourselves in. We have mistaken beliefs in organizations and follow paths that promise unimaginable outcomes. Cryptocurrency is one of the numberless ones that come to my mind. We also think that things will be static, that our situations will always be the same. This is delusion too, as we learn nothing stays the same. Or we think that if we get that house, job, spouse, child, or whatever, it will change who we are. Make us happy. We fail to realize that chasing after things proves to be an empty endeavor. And then, we try again. Commonly this can be called insanity: doing the same thing, expecting something different. We can maybe hear our delusion when we think, oh, the grass is greener over there. It may be for a time. It doesn't last. Each place you go, you take yourself with you.

This is insight into delusion, but it isn't to say we should accept unacceptable conditions or remain in a mindset of depraved resolve. No, being aware of delusions requires that we see what we're going after and why, and are attentive to the possibility of our not seeing clearly—which we aren't, since that's the nature of being, and all acts and intents are conditioned, which in turn have outcomes, clouding our vision until we experience them. Greed, hate and anger, and delusion provide us with the foundation of suffering. This is the human condition; this is what we're always trying to escape.

The Four Noble Truths and the Noble Eightfold Path

Like clouds in the sky, memories, dreams, hopes, wants, and expectations come and go. Does anyone actually get what they want and remain satisfied with it? Or is there the thought, "Oh, I thought it was going to be different." Does anyone remember the past as it was? You have your version of the story, and others have theirs. Somewhere they say, in between, there lies the truth. We want to be right so that our truth supports our point of view, which is grounded in greed, hate and anger, and delusion. These are again wrapped in getting, desire, wanting, and grasping. Craving. Here is basically where the Buddha's *Four Noble Truths* come in. There is suffering in this world. Everyone suffers. Desire is the cause of suffering. Releasing desires is the way out of suffering, and following the *Noble Eightfold Path* can get us off the cycle of causes and conditions, life and death.

Everyone is suffering. I'm suffering, your friends, people you interact with everywhere are suffering too. Everyone is suffering since life on earth is uncertain, death is always just there. Just answer this question or ask it: Is what you have or what you're experiencing what you want or wanted? What you expected? Almost always the answer is well, not exactly. And for us who have a lived experience and history within antiblack racism, we have deeply rooted "we're not loved or wanted" by the overarching social structure and we moreover have been told directly and indirectly that we don't belong in it. In one way or another, the social ills that we experience, such as poverty or poor health, substandard housing or education, and so on, stem in part from the insistence on the rhetoric and messages that come from that deep place. Graciously, we don't have to stay there. Realization that everyone is suffering is one of the keys to dancing away from these mental constructs. Just think of the others who have conditions that cause them pain. Immigrants at the borders, people sitting in the midst of wars, those with no water systems. Or those who can't trust anyone due to always feeling afraid, those who are greedy, hoarding more wealth than could ever be spent even if they underwrote basic incomes for everyone. I know, you may think having lots of money will solve your position in life. While it may, what it won't solve is an ego attachment generating anger and self-focus. What's important is to know deeply that each time we resolve we're in any given situation resulting from antiblack racism, we merely reinforce it in our minds, abandoning the opportunity to change it from the inside. And instead we think something or someone "out there" should change so we can feel better. The Buddha had an awareness of an answer to the why, and the way out of suffering. These are called *the Four Noble Truths* of Suffering and were the main teachings that came out of the Buddha's Awakening.[1]

The Four Noble Truths of Suffering

There is suffering
There is a cause of suffering
There is freedom from suffering
There is a Path of Liberation from Suffering

It's pretty simple and easy to concur that yes, there is suffering. We suffer as soon as we get what we want or have what we don't want. It could be a feeling of lack, such as we don't have a material object, or satisfying relationships, or certain children, or a job. These are external objects we aspire to have. And, of course, in the United States, the economy is built upon getting things and putting together and keeping the American Dream. Even if you don't buy into or deny the American Dream, the beat of consumption and buying is very strong. It may be shrouded in watching television programing or making sure you get what you're looking for, that is, the best deal.

These desires are often the basis for scams. You know, there are people out there full of greed, anger, and delusion, happy to separate us from our cash by telling us a tall tale. And much of the time we fall for the tale when we do, clinging to what we want or desire. Our society is a society of "more" and "not enough." Look at people standing in lines the day after Thanksgiving. I'm not saying having a good life is undesirable; I'm saying the Buddha said desire is the source of suffering.

Desires are forever morphing, changing, evolving; therefore we unconsciously see that everything is impermanent. Nothing lasts. The first feeling of good always disappears eventually. So we try to repeat it, relive it, in different ways maybe. Even though we can't always see the change, it's changing anyway. Me, you, the computer systems, friends, animals, trees, mountains, the ocean. That impermanence is at the base, driving desire. We want to keep the thrill going, not look at death, try to grasp and hold on to something. Of course there are people, places, situations, and things we want to change that don't appear to. That's desire as well!

Therefore, basically, the cause of suffering is wanting, or desire, and for innumerable times it's based on wanting to feel good or at least not feel bad. This is the Second Noble Truth. Feeling good comes through the five senses: sight, sound, scent, taste, and touch. We can add to this, that feeling good also comes through mental and emotional states. Being respected, having enough money, belonging, and being loved for who we are regardless of whatever. Mental and emotional states are what drive the ego. It's also where we find separation, that is, we feel distant from people or that we think what we do doesn't affect them. Each time we go through the cycle of wanting, getting, believing we are separate, losing the feeling of being loved, and wanting again, we suffer.[2] And at first, realizing this happens innumerable times a day can be overwhelming. At the bottom of the suffering is fear caused by impermanence inherent in life in general: that at some point we know we and everyone will die, we will no longer be in this body and have this mind. We don't know why.

Freedom from suffering, the Third Noble Truth, comes from relinquishing desire, relinquishing fear, and being okay with and accepting impermanence. Know that death is a part of living. No amount of anything will ever change that fact. Here we can stop clinging to ideas that drive us to want more. We can take a moment to see what our ego is doing, running us into the ground with cravings. See how we are conditioned by external messages or causes, that drive us to do certain things. You may think, what kind of life will I have if I desire nothing? Certainly, if your life is nonjudgmental, nongrasping, and accepting through the practice of these and other realizations, there is peace and ease. That means you live your true life fully, live your life differently than you've been conditioned with. And that's a joy in and of itself. How do we do this? That's the Fourth Noble Truth: Follow the path of liberation. This path is called *the Noble Eightfold Path.*

The Noble Eightfold Path of Liberation from Suffering

Instead of living in fear of impermanence, and being driven by desire, we live in compassion. We make promises, or vows, that we can keep by putting others first, and finding our way out of the traps of antiblack racism as it has defined us knowingly or unknowingly. We need, as the Buddha outlined, eight interconnecting and intertwining aspects of behaving and thinking.

The Right View
The Right Intention
The Right Action
The Right Speech
The Right Livelihood
The Right Effort
The Right Mindfulness
The Right Meditation

The Right View takes into consideration the basis for existence, which for the Buddha included knowing and dealing with impermanence, realizing that this life is suffering and why it's suffering, and understanding that there isn't an independent self. Everyone's life is supported by everyone else, which means the ego can be transformed. With ego transformation, enlightenment can be seen where you're standing.

And Right Intention gets at our thinking, motivations, and actions. When we talk about ego, we're talking about relinquishing selfishness, self-centeredness, and seeing instead interdependence upon every aspect of this world. This helps us to have that critical appropriate response that's not about me so much, that the Buddha spoke of, and being compassionate with others as well as our selves. Here we do our best to move in a stream of generosity, love, and kindness, and we are being and acting in attentive reality. Right Action on the Noble Eightfold Path means avoiding doing things that are deemed unloving and hurtful to self and others. Not killing, and not taking things that aren't offered, are examples. Also, abstaining from ingesting or selling drugs and alcohol or other intoxicants falls here. Taking Right Action includes moderation and healthy choices in eating, as well as having a moderate relationship with social media and consumer involvement. Thich Nhat Hanh suggested that we turn off all media, stop watching violent and sexually abusive programs, and reduce our talking topics to those that are wholesome (Hanh, 2002). Doing these reduces anger and aggression, greed, and delusion. Not only that, also engaging with sexual acts only in wholesome circumstances is part and parcel to Right Action.

Right Speech is the next area of the Noble Eightfold Path. Please keep in mind these areas are not stages; they occur simultaneously. In order to explain them, we take them one at a time. How you say what you say is as important as what you say. In what and how we say something, we can reveal our true thoughts. Sarcasm, passive aggressiveness, making inappropriate jokes, and even keeping silence when saying something is needed can violate the spirit of Right Speech. Here, think of what needs to be said, when it should be said and why. Does what you say benefit or hurt? Of course, when we determine something needs to be said, it may not go over well. Are you speaking from love or criticism? What is your intention in saying something? Is it for your relief or to help the other person? In this arena, we also avoid gossip and argumentation, lying, or puffing ourselves up at the expense of another.

How do we earn a living? This is where Right Livelihood comes in. Do you help people with the work you do? Does your work help reduce or eliminate suffering? Can you balance your life and living needs as you also work? Can compassion and kindness be the driving force for your living? Are you only focused on making money? Getting ahead? Achieving? If so, that's the opposite of Right Livelihood. There's nothing wrong with learning a skill or being good at something or doing a job well so that Right Livelihood can be had. Truly, anything that earns money for you that hurts others, and puts yourself first and above them, or comes from greed, hate and anger, or delusion, should be closely examined.

Effort is the next right thing we'll talk about. Right Effort means not going to extremes in anything while mixing Right Action with Right Intention in honor of being freed from suffering. This involves doing what is necessary to be moderate in eating, keeping from intoxicants for yourself and others, keeping yourself from unwholesome sexual engagements, and spending time in meditation. We'll get to meditation in a moment; I did say these aspects of the path are not linear, remember? Right Effort is what's needed for ongoing practice and realization of enlightenment. Noticing and attending to thoughts like "I don't want to do..." or "I don't feel like doing..." or "I want what I want..." increases and supports Right Effort. It's frequently about doing the right thing when you don't want to do it anyway until you *want* to do the right thing. Aid comes to you too when you "just do it." By doing that, new habit patterns are formed and before you know it, old patterns are dropped and freedom from suffering emerges.

I talked a bit already in a different chapter about the mindfulness market. Here though, Right Mindfulness isn't about trying to sell an enlightenment experience to someone for profit and gain. Yes, employers are selling mindfulness to employees so that they can be more productive. Many companies offer apps and programs that are intended to help you be more mindful. Know deeply for sure, mindfulness is a central part of Buddhist practice and can't be abstracted out like separating yolks from whites of eggs. Mindfulness is being attentive at every moment, putting others first, being present with what you're doing. So when someone says, we have to be mindful of what we say, for example, it means we are thinking of the entirety of what causes suffering and how to reduce it before we respond with words, thoughts, or body language or actions. If you're sitting there reading your phone and there are people around for dinner, are you present? Attentive? Are you thinking of yourself? When you're dwelling on thoughts, are you being mindful or are you thinking of the past and the future? Are you giving yourself fully to what is arising in the moment, whether it's work, or listening to a lecture, or cleaning up a spill? Right mindfulness is being here, being here now, in the present, attentive. Not letting the mind wander off, being aware and supportive of others, not all about self.

This brings us to Right Meditation. Meditation is also as charged as mindfulness. There are meditation apps and all sorts of stuff you can buy to help you meditate. I have no issue with that; just in this Zen Buddhist practice that you're reading about, we practice Zazen, which I'll cover with details in Chapter 3. For now, meditation is a way to focus your mind to calm your breathing, to slow down to recognize life as it is. Some people do meditation to get something from it, such as a lower heart rate, to reduce stress or suffering or to get a perspective, or slow the trigger to anger time. It can be done with the eyes open or closed. It can be guided or unguided. Types of meditation are numerous and they come from many different paths. For Zen Buddhists, we sit in Zazen, without seeking for anything at all, not expecting anything.

As we practice the Buddha's Eightfold Path and place and keep our attention on the noble truths of suffering, we are able to now focus on emptiness and what that means for letting go of ego and self.

Emptiness and Impermanence

Emptiness in simple terms is a description. It means there is no "you" or "me" that exists "separately from" others. We only exist in relation to other people, animals, mountains, rivers, oceans, and a world held together by a universe. This is called dependent co-arising. The concept of "this then that," or "not this and therefore not that," underlies dependent co-origination.

In other words, causes and conditions arise based on our interactions with others, the world, and the universe. Often it's stated as "if this, then that" or "if not this, then not that."

We depend on others for our very living experience. If there were

no folks cultivating food, we wouldn't have food. If no one was providing homes to live in, we would have nowhere to live. All the pieces
and parts of food and housing, as well as our bodies, come from the
elements: water, air, earth. We can't live without animals or trees
or reproduction. We are interconnected, in other words. When you
examine phenomena, you find that it's all that way. Nothing can exist
on its own. Therefore, there isn't anything graspable, to our chagrin,
that makes us "a Self" or makes something "an Other." Nothing is
graspable and everything is changing. That everything is changing is
the Zen Buddhist term for impermanence in our constructed world.
The constructed world is that world around us, which includes the
construction of antiblack racism. Antiblack racism isn't graspable. It
is an idea that needs your interdependence for it to exist. It doesn't
exist separately from you or other people and it is empty.

Even if we can't detect change or the impermanence going on with
the human consciousness, still everything is changing. Grasping at
thinking it's not changing and that we are separate from it is affirming
the self and ego. Affirming the self is affirming ego, and affirming ego
is therefore affirming duality, the separation between you and me, the
valuing of one object over another. Moving away from grasping and
toward realizing emptiness means we don't have to depend on constructed concepts like me and my, versus you and yours, which affirm
the ego and solidify separation in order to exist. And where there is a
deconstructed and examined released ego that used to justify a position, a set of beliefs, or a want, "no self" can arise—stated differently,
Buddha Nature can be realized. This means we can think about the
world we live in as not so much one in which we are powerless over, or
victims in, or not wanted in, or have to hold on to so tightly in delusion. Everyone is wanted, loved, and supported in Buddha Nature.

Powerfulness is a desire to control, which underpins racial
structures, and really establishes the *I versus you*, or the *us versus
them, who has and who doesn't*. All the way down to me being told
to "get off the car" when I was a child, to the control witnessed in
Apartheid. Those who perceive themselves as having no power often
blame those that they perceive do have power. With power structures, there comes the control of the distribution of resources, the

setting up of the ego, the reinforcement of casting the other off, or oppressing them. My childhood compadre appeared oppressive, the board member who demanded that I not do a certain thing was exacting her concept of power, and Elon Musk makes huge use of power to control people.

So, when there is no powerfulness, there is no lack of power, or powerlessness arises in the form of realization of emptiness. If you think of an example of when you felt powerlessness, and trace it back to how your ego was involved, your desire for something, you'll see and be able to let it go. At that point you'll also be able to see that what you wanted was based on some kind of grasping that caused suffering. Or maybe you have a belief in a cultural situation that has you thinking you *should have* received or been treated a certain way. That attaches to your ego and not being aware of that attachment, and you suffer by believing perceptions that cause your sadness and anger. We can look easily at relationships in our families or at work to see this at play. I want my family, for example, to acknowledge my accomplishments. That's my ego. When they don't, I get mad. That's my ego. Why do I want them to acknowledge my accomplishments? It's only truly from the fact that I aspire to receive a ton of fame or power. I know I'm not alone in this aspiration. Where does that desire come from? Somewhere outside of me, arising from constructed social norms or feelings of lack, or from trying to hold on to and prevent constant change.

Rather than live by the constraints of power and grasping onto that which is impermanent and always changing and can't exist on its own without others, it may be conducive to not only realize the truth and path of elimination of suffering. It is also very important to live by wisdom and compassion, which are developed through what are known as *the Wisdom Paramitas.*

The Wisdom Paramitas

Like the Noble Eightfold Path, the *Wisdom Paramitas*, which when realized and practiced are considered to be perfections in our characters leading to wisdom, are described independently for the purpose of understanding them. They overlap just as aspects of the Noble Eightfold Path do. Reliance on the *Wisdom Paramitas* is to bring you to the point of wisdom, where there isn't so much adherence to constructed ideas, the ability to be attentive, and to see causes and conditions arising. While the *Wisdom Paramitas* are given originally in Sanskrit, here I will state them very simply in English. They are generosity, personal ethical conduct, patience, effort and perseverance, mental concentration, and wisdom.

What I really love about the *Wisdom Paramitas* is that I can get close to intentionality and apply a different view that sets aside my ego. Starting with generosity, ask the question, what am I giving? Then ask yourself, why am I giving? There is a three-sided triangular notion that giving requires a giver, recipient, and a gift. A lot of times, in our social world, a gift from a giver has a string attached. We give presents for different occasions, or we give donations for causes. Maybe we want to have reciprocity for the presents or acknowledgment of our charitable donation engraved on a wall or something. Those are gifts with strings attached. The receiver is aware of the string in many cases, so they don't always reciprocate. In situations where we give, though, the strings aren't so obvious. Perhaps we think if I give this gift, they'll like me or they'll contract with my firm. Monetary and material gifts with strings known or unknown are often what comes to mind when we talk about generosity. It doesn't have to be that way, and this *Paramita* supports knowing what you're giving and why. If there's a string, acknowledge it. You can also give with no strings. To do so, you have to carefully think about it before you do the deed. Alongside the tangible, intangible gifts abound, like kind speech or giving appreciation or gratitude for someone's efforts. If these are given without strings— I'm not praising the person to get them to do something for me, or to acknowledge me—they are equal to and in some cases far more skillful than a material gift. Think about your giving, the gift, and the recipient of the gift before you give. I used to think that material gifts were best. I don't think that anymore. Appreciably, I see where my ego gets involved and avoid grasping for any kind of praise, recognition, acknowledgment. Think giving of self for benefiting and providing merit for others, secretly, and not having a desire for anyone to know about the gift.

Personal ethics comprises the *Paramita* containing conduct, morality, and discipline. How we behave in thinking, speaking, and acting is the overarching concern. It's putting attentiveness on everything we do, think and say. Here we can get our arms around our own behaviors, and find ways to be temperate in what we used to allow impulsively, such as through addiction, carelessness, or other unskillful acts and lack of concern for how we impact the people we are in this reality with. It's about doing the right actions on the Noble Eightfold Path without being conflicted about doing those right actions and knowing the right action causes no harm. Setting aside time to meditate consistently, acting compassionately especially in situations that make us angry, keeping one's word, stopping thinking about someone we are resentful toward—these are examples of personal ethics.

Next we address patience with everything and everyone, and everyone includes ourselves. Being patient means knowing that pushing too hard or too fast doesn't bring an end to suffering. We reduce the love we have for anger, and can go through life with a sense of equanimity, not easily upset or frustrated at everything that doesn't go the way we want it to. Patience also allows imperfection, which as humans we all experience and suffer through. Decidedly, I think it helps us drop the adherence to being right even when we feel we are, like when we want to say, "I told you so." Or getting upset when someone we love chooses a not so comfortable way of life that may also bring us discomfort.

Effort and perseverance are just that. Put the appropriate time, energy, and thought into something and keep at it. Don't give up when it gets harder than you expected. Give up procrastination and giving into feelings of "I don't feel like it" or "I don't want to." It's easy to see that the ego is driving those feelings and thoughts when recognizing it's used to getting you to do what it wants, rather than what would be beneficial to everyone. Your thinking is to be about helping others, and the limitlessness of helping others requires effort and perseverance. Consider the person who is constantly lying or who won't visit a medical person in spite of the clear need. Or the person who constantly indulges in substances or who is hurtful by the way they speak. Now, this isn't to say that you have to condone unskillful behavior or stay in a situation that isn't beneficial. You do have the choice. To be able to use effort and perseverance will lead you closer to the wisdom you need to make or accept any changes.

The last two *Wisdom Paramitas* are mental concentration and wisdom. Mentally concentrating and being focused is the key to being attentive in the now. You don't get overwhelmed by your mind taking you down tangents and riding on hamster wheels. You're not beating yourself up or imagining some oasis where life has no changing landscape. You can listen to people in your life and be there for them to help them. You're not self-obsessed or self-absorbed to their exclusion. You sit Zazen regularly and have nothing to gain. It's just sitting. And with the previous *Wisdom Paramitas* wisdom arises. You can see clearly what reality is and what delusion does. You're aware of delusion and doing your best to be mindful. Wisdom helps us navigate through the codependent origination that comes with this life, the causes and conditions that arise from what we do or don't do. We can see how our lives are contingent on how we interact with people, ideas, and objects in the world. And indeed we can behave in ways that provide a great benefit to everyone and take ourselves off the center of the universe. Let go deeply.

Together with the *Wisdom Paramitas*, we also live by vow. We have these perfections of generosity, personal ethics, patience, perseverance, mental fortitude, and wisdom. These help us relieve our egos, pointing us to living by vow.

Living by Vow

In Buddhism, there is a concept, which I mentioned, of if this, then that. Some call that causes and conditions; some call it karma. Karma is a term that relates to causes and effects. Many volumes exist on the subject of karma, so many that it's not something I delve into here. After all, being unaware of causes and conditions, or "if this, then that," can lead us to being driven by greed, hate and anger, and delusion. Incorporating the *Wisdom Paramitas* and living by vow breaks us free from being unaware of or inattentive to causes and conditions. Rather, we live by intentionality and promises and avowing. They are the conglomeration or the amalgamation of the Noble Eightfold Path and the *Wisdom Paramitas* in the Zen Buddhist path.

What are these vows? Generally known as the *Bodhisattva Precepts*, simply stated, they are promises to live in a way that benefits all beings, not to be self-centered, and help us to keep our attention on enlightenment. Enlightenment isn't something that arises in the future. It is here now; we just have to know it in our hearts. First, we start with overarching vows, promising to refrain from all evil, and then to make every effort to live in enlightenment, and then finally, to live for and be living to benefit all beings. Then, we delve deeper. We promise to honor life, and to not take what's not given. We vow to be honorable in sexuality, and to refrain from saying false words. Refraining from giving, receiving, or selling intoxicating substances and to not put other people down are the next two vows we make. Then, we agree to not be self-aggrandizing or greedy, or to hold onto resentments or hatred and anger toward someone or something. When we make a mistake, we avow influences that push us to live outside the precepts.

When we live this way rather than in the culturally conditioned way, our ego isn't driving us. Our suffering is lessened. We get to see Buddha Dharma and reality right before us. This provides a refuge for our minds and bodies to bathe in as we make decisions and take actions in living.

The Sixteen Bodhisattva Vows

These vows contain what are known as the Refuges, the Pure Precepts, and Ten Grave Precepts (Anderson, 2001; Baker, 2023). Please know that these are not to be read as "I have to do these perfectly to be good" with rigid adherence (Baker, 2023). No, no, not at all. They are to be incorporated into the ways of moving through life, incorporated into the *Wisdom Paramitas*. Living these vows fluidly helps to realize the *Four Noble Truths* and the *Noble Eightfold Path*. You can find them like this or slightly modified, depending on where you practice.

The Refuges (or Recurrently Known as the Three Treasures)

- I take refuge in Buddha before all beings, immersing body and mind deeply in the Way, awakening true mind.
- I take refuge in Dharma before all beings, entering deeply the merciful ocean of Buddha's Way.
- I take refuge in Sangha before all beings, bringing harmony to everyone, free from hindrance.

Three Pure Precepts

- I vow to refrain from all evil.
- I vow to make every effort to live in enlightenment.
- I vow to live and be lived for the benefit of all beings.

Ten Grave Precepts

1. I vow not to kill.
2. I vow not to take what isn't given.
3. I vow not to misuse sexuality.
4. I vow to refrain from false speech.
5. I vow to refrain from intoxicants.
6. I vow not to slander.
7. I vow not to praise self at the expense of others.
8. I vow not to be avaricious.
9. I vow not to harbor ill will.
10. I vow not to disparage the Three Treasures.

Buddhism for American Blacks

Earlier in the book, I suggested that when interacting with racially impacted people in the United States, what arises from the lack of power belief system is an immediate concretization of the ego, with a systematic blame of the other for the predicament, situation, life position, and ugliness that life presented them. Marvin Gaye sings about how it makes him "want to holler" the way they do his life.[3] Appreciation is granted for the music and the way it inspired, recognizing at the same time that it was rife with blaming in many cases.

In a so-called racialized society, which it appears that many societies are to one degree or another, when the individual buys into the idea that they are inferior or believes that the powerful have dominion over them, they are immediately cast in a victim role, and therefore see the Other as the perpetrator, preventing them from getting what they want. Thus, within those same social structures, the racialized group interferes with its own ability to realize powerlessness and ego removal are the way out. Of course, no one wants to blame the victim since that's not appropriate. Just the same, it's deluded, greedy, angry, and fearful thinking that causes the suffering with the focus on the self, the lack of understanding of what the self really is. Simply stated, this requires looking inward with the attention to the *Wisdom Paramitas* and springing from our vows to respond, and not expecting people out there to change, not demanding to be compensated from the belief that it's owed. We refrain from taking what's not given as one of our promises. This requires turning inside and developing a way to watch thinking and seeing where it leads.

As a thought arises, an emotion comes with it. Emotions aren't facts, and if one can see through and trace back to the thought that leads to the emotion, which stirs the ego, and intervene on one's behalf, change can occur. That process really helped me! And now lately, an interesting exercise has been to try to remove *I, me, my, mine*—any possessive stance as if something, including emotions, belonged to me—from speech, writing, thinking, and judging. When bothered by an event, such as a person on the road cuts in front of me and I get angry, or why I didn't receive a contract I wanted, trying to evaluate where the anger originates and how it comes from ego, wanting fame and gain really, it helps to let it pass while being uninvolved. I liken this to watching a stream flowing down the street with debris in it. I'd never pick up the trash! When feeling down and sad as feelings arise from the way that labels of brown and the ability to birth children are applied to this body, and the treatment it receives, the looks it gets, trying to see it as just a thing flowing by, just this, is a great practice to engage in this way. Let the conditioned response of retaliation, rebellion, anger, and resentment or even trying to explain how difference makes no sense arise. Then move through that without grasping on the "why" of the treatment. Remember, there is no separation. The need instead is for compassion and realization that all are conditioned structures. These steps cool the situation. This isn't to suggest that skillful words aren't said, or skillful action isn't taken. They are. It's just to say that here's a way to trace feelings and to stop them from dictating actions. Herein lie powerfulness and emptiness, living by the *Wisdom Paramitas* and vows, acknowledging Buddha Nature.

To summarize ways of living the Zen Buddhist path for American Blacks, please know that the locus of control over your mind is inside you, and we are living in a collective codependent world. We need each other, can't live without each other or the flora and fauna of the earth. Greed, hate and anger, and delusion cause racist issues. Following the *Four Noble Truths* into the *Noble Eightfold Path* and then into the *Wisdom Paramitas* provides the way out of desire and a release of ego. These allow us to put others first, and put our egos aside. As we live day to day by vows and avowals, remember everything is constantly changing and that nothing is self-created.

3

Zen Buddhist Movement and Dance Meditation

Going beyond reveals real miracles in nothing special
moves in thusness—Tanahashi, 2013, p. 287

In this chapter, I briefly share with you how dance is a deep practice of meditation, how it's used therapeutically, and embodying Zen Buddhist forms as dances. I'll go about this in a very direct manner I hope, pointing out some research on dance and its effectiveness in working with diseases, as well as the way dance has been shown to communicate through an indirect pathway to get us hooked on buying products and services. After that, I turn to describe the Buddha's Awakening and the Bodhisattva path. Once that's covered, I go into aspects of birth and death from a Zen Buddhist perspective as I understand it. Within that context, cause and effect and enlightenment arise as topics. Then, I encourage supporting yourselves and your arousal of enlightenment with a daily practice and finding and working with a transmitted Dharma teacher.

Dance as Nonverbal, Nondiscursive, and Nondual

The fact that we move our bodies is given. There're many activities included in movement, such as walking, running, hiking, climbing, cycling, skiing, court games and field games, and working out at the gym. Let's not forget social dancing, where we dance and have a good time. In addition, we can't leave out yoga, tai chi, qigong, and many other ways of moving to connect with the essence of the body and mind. What happens with the dropping away of focus on the self is amazing when engaged with the awe-producing aspects of movement. The feeling of vastness and a reprieve in letting go of all thoughts, worries, concerns, and problems take over. If you happen to be dancing in company of other people, you form a nondiscursive and bodily connection with them. Indeed, we have this experience lots of times when we dance, as well as when we simply watch dance (Walter, 2015).

Dance is a metaphor, too, for lots of actions that we can't quite describe in words. We say, "my mind danced when I saw that," or to describe a relationship, we may say, "we're in this dance together," or we might also say, "you're dancing around the topic." It's from intuition that we know the way that dance operates, and saying these kinds of relational phrases makes our meaning clear. Like Buddha Dharma, dance is beyond words. Yes, you can actually describe a dance if you're able to articulate each movement. In the academic dance world, different systems of notation attempt to do this. Don't worry, I'm not talking about creating or relying on a notation system. I'm focused on the nondiscursive aspects of dance and other movements, what they communicate, and how they get at our essence and expressions.

Our First Nations People danced. From the Africans to the Australians, since very much before the Common Era, history has documented the inclusion of dance and what I term sacred dance (Walter 2020). This type of dance was part and parcel of daily life, in rituals, in transitions, in healing and in celebrations. Importantly as well, the ancestors in these nations used dance as spiritual practice to connect with Dharma: in other words, a way of knowing to drop away the body and mind, to create connections and awareness of our position on the planet with other sentient and insentient beings, and within the known and unknown universes. It's what I call *Dance Dharma*, or Dancing No Self, or Dance as Buddha Nature, and that applies to each form of dance and movement where the focus on the self, the body, and the mind drops away. It's a point of departure from duality. In a previous chapter I talked about duality: the sense of opposites. Up and down, left and right, right and wrong, male and female, good and bad. Duality gives us the way for creating likes and dislikes, judgments, comparative dimensions, and so on. We need duality in walking around on the earth; sadly, until someone brings it to our attention in a way we can comprehend it, we don't necessarily immediately see how duality can make or break us, keep us locked in creating causes and conditions that may be unfavorable or unskillful. Perhaps you might argue that dance movement is the opposite of stillness. I ask you to consider stillness as movement, a concentration on breathing and attentiveness that has its own action and level of awe. When the body is still, we might be able to detect the movement of the lungs or the dance of digestion or feel the actioned heartbeat. So there is a great deal of movement when we're still.

Dance Impacts the Body and Mind

When you see or do dancing, how do you respond? For many people, we are drawn to mesmerized or hypnotic states. Whether you think you can dance or whether you know you can, it's a natural phenomenon to stare at it with awe. The way that dance impacts the body and mind has informed an entire certified and therapeutic field of study using dance. One way dance movement therapy (DMT) is practiced comes through the American Dance Therapy Association. DMT often employs a dance therapist at a medical institution or in a professional office or can be accessed via online videos or books. Dance therapy programs offer ways to deal with organ cancers, such as breast cancers. One dance therapy article connected dance with pain management, and concluded pain was reduced with dance and as a physical practice it may improve quality of life (Cruz et al., 2022). The article's authors call for studies and clinical trials that integrate dance as adjuvant therapy in cancer treatments. Whether at home, online, or at the theater, a dance club, or other social venue, dancing for well-being isn't limited to clinical applications by a trained therapist.

Dance doing or watching takes us out of the head space and into the heart, to that ephemeral place of wholeness and connection to humanity. It's a meditation practice that is unsurpassed. It works on our brains and our bodies. We can dance while sitting or lying down or watch or imagine dance and receive great benefits. Though dance has yet to be shown to cure bodily malfunctions, dance doing supports protocols for treatment of health conditions and contributes to well-being and quality of life.

For example, research on dance and Alzheimer's disease confirms dance's effectiveness on physical and cognitive function, functionality, psychological outcomes, and quality of life in people with the disease (Ruiz-Muelle & Lópe-Rodriguez, 2019). Also, for Parkinson's disease it's been reported that dance is a nonpharmacological, effective, affordable, and engaging intervention for dealing with that disease. And dance interventions positively impact global cognition, memory, and balance, and significantly reduce depression (Tao et al., 2023). When it comes to cancer, in the article "Effect of Dance on Cancer-Related Fatigue and Quality of Life," the authors found significant improvements for cancer-related fatigue and suggested that dance might be an effective treatment for it (Sturm et al., 2014).

Dance is also a connector to consumer behaviors, attachment to products and services.

Just by watching dance you can be influenced if it's connected to something (Walter, 2015). Relative to cancer treatment, a preliminary conclusion was that watching dance in a theater improved bodily strength, emotional relief, and personal agency, and increased self-esteem (Weis et al., 2022).

Dance as Meditation

And dance done as meditation practice provides a nonverbal prediscursive place in our bodies and minds that supports release of tension, stress, and anxiety. "The movement of the body through various physical activities increases special neurotransmitter substances in the brain (endorphins) which creates a state of well-being.

3. Zen Buddhist Movement and Dance Meditation

Body movements through dance enhance the body's physical functions (circulatory, respiratory, skeletal, and muscular systems), including also mental and emotional well-being of the person. Dance is found to reduce stress and anxiety, creates greater self-awareness and boosts self-esteem" (Thiagarajan & Mokhtar, 2022, p. 43).

In a 2020 study, the importance of dance meditation was discussed within a

> connection between body movements and the nervous system, highlighting the neuronal correlates of dance recently evidenced by new methods in neuroscience of dance, showing how dance can positively act on the brain and the nerves and opening a wide range of opportunities to deal with body-mind health based in therapeutic dance approaches. ... recent methods allow demonstrating the therapeutic benefits of different dance approaches, that appear closely related to the essential role of body consciousness promoted by dancing (1) ... In addition to the brain plasticity, dance also largely affects the plasticity of the spinal cord and peripheral nerves throughout the rest of the body [Gomes et al., 2021, p. 6].

It is important to note the impact and effect these authors saw on the spinal cord, where MM often takes hold and hostages the body. In my experience, gentle movements of the spine have aided the reduction of pain and the flexibility of my spine.

Dance meditation brings up the True Self, so to speak, through intentional and unintentional movements. It travels outside of words. I've coined the term *Theodance*—any dance that connects with the mystical meanings and experiences of human beings. It's a nonverbal discourse on the sacred. *Theodance* gives us the ability to share intuitive and sacred knowledge through mystical meanings and experiences contained in the dance. Engaging with *Theodance* contributes to a planetary spiritual movement, increases well-being, and provides a stabilizing force. It's a universal language and communication vehicle like no other, connecting somatically and neurologically, intuitively and instinctively. A *Theodance* mystical experience occurs on a continuum, from having fun to the experience of transcendence and immanence. Dance provides a way for us to find strength in those all-too-important aspects. It builds on itself, builds confidence in our choices. It assures us that we're loved and cared for and that this day-to-day existence isn't all that is happening. And it doesn't matter what the dance looks like or what type it is. It gives us moments to focus on something beautiful and allows us to turn off our thinking, worrying, and fears.

Buddhists and Dance

Practicing Buddhists have danced many dances, as was pointed out by the anthropologist Joan Erdman. Also,

> [There are] three terms that are very helpful in appreciating essential aspects of dance in Buddhism: dance actual, dance depicted, and dance ephemeral. When Buddhist dance is seen to manifest in each of these realms, its full potency as a medium of religion and spiritual practice becomes clearer. ... Buddhist dance can be understood as something multi-dimensional, transformative, and consciousness-altering. By understanding these three aspects of Buddhist dance—actual, depicted, and ephemeral—its full meaning is easier to grasp and the reason for its prominence in art makes more sense. Placing dance in a mandala: depicted, visualized, or actualized, further strengthens the correspondence between dance and the practice of mystical Buddhism [Houseal, 2020].

Buddhist dancing often happens after an insight into the entirety of one's life. For example, one of the Buddha's main disciples, Mogallana, "danced for joy." After his mother transitioned from birth and death, he realized that she was the Bodhisattva that had led him to the Buddhist path (Kusunoki, 2002). I'll have more to say about birth and death, and what it means to be a *Bodhisattva*, someone who helps others, a bit later in the chapter.

For the moment, consider dance meditation as an aspect of mindfulness concentration as described in the *Wisdom Paramitas*. By incorporating movement into meditation, Buddhist practitioners deepen their awareness of the present moment, and cultivate nonseparation within the Buddha World. In my view, some dance meditations have been incorporated into the sacred movements carried out as part of developing this aspect of realizing nonseparation.

These include bowing, walking, and mudra postures, as well as moving with intentionality when moving throughout space. Some are included as *forms*, or ways to move in the practice, and others are included or subsumed vows and interacting with others. Forms are what we do as we dance through space as part of honoring the Buddhas and Ancestors. Forms also provide us with those nondual aspects of dance meditation that allow us to let go of conditioned responses and ways of being, to let go of ourselves.

Here I start with bowing, then I'll go into *Kinhin* or walking, and the mudras associated with what I call Dance Dharma, or Dance as Buddha Nature for Zen Buddhists.

Bowing and Gassho

Bowing is a very spiritual practice in Zen Buddhism and I categorized it as a Dance Dharma. A bow is a way of being respectful, of acknowledging each other, and sharing the profound path of awakening. It's also a way to honor ancestors and teachers. Bows are done when passing someone on a path, when sitting down to eat, when beginning Zazen, during certain ceremonies, when needing forgiveness, and at many other times. Bows are also a form of greeting, when both encountering and leaving someone's presence. Embodying longer and shorter durations for bows can transmit inner intentions. Holding a bow for more than just a second or two is probably a skillful way to convey that you acknowledge the person or group you're encountering. A really long bow for more than a few seconds conveys deep respect and honor to the recipient of your bow. Often, the bows are reciprocated, but depending on the situation or the place, they may be received by the other person with them holding *Gassho*. Three different types of bows come into play: standing bows, floor bows or prostrations, and seated bows.

In doing a standing bow, habitually, people bend forward at the waist if their back is strong! If not, they bend more from the knees by bending them some and leaning forward with the spine straight if the back can't handle a forward bend, or you can bend more from the hips. In this bend you have to keep your back straight. If the back or hips can't handle a forward bend, you can bend from the neck slightly. In practicing the forms, many times there are bells or other sounds taking place to let you know when to bow and when to stand.

Floor bows are bows completed by touching the knees and then the forehead to the floor. You follow the same flow as with a standing bow I just mentioned. Here, as you bend forward you bend the knees, fold at the hips, place the arms down to steady yourself, and touch the head to the floor, or the cushion if one is there. While there, we lift our palms up by our ears.[1] Then you reverse the movements to return to standing.

Seated bows are just that, you bend forward from the hips slightly, or lower your head.

Who or what do we bow to? This is different for many people. In the beginning we bow to gratitude for being shown a peaceful way to live. Maybe we bow to the fact that we are here to help others, and maybe that we bow to appreciate that we aren't alone on the earth. We bow then to the earth, the ocean, the sky for what they do for our life. We bow to our ancestors, parents, and children for all they have given us. We bow to get our ego out of our way, appreciating humility. Eventually we also bow to Shakyamuni Buddha, Buddhas and Ancestors, the Dharma, and the Sangha. We bow to everything and everyone for being there to help us in our short lives to realize delusion and enlightenment.

Make no mistake, though: Bowing isn't "worshiping idols" as one might be led to construe it as. In the Christian doctrines people are admonished severely to avoid such a practice. Bowing isn't a representation of god or an object of worship, it isn't a physical object. It doesn't represent a devotional image. Rather, bowing is a state of mind, a reverence and respect for the importance of your attentiveness and that of others, the planet and the universe.

During a bow, the hands are placed in a particular position. Place both palms together at the mid-sternum area, with the fingers held together, and pointing upward. Your wrists come close to the body, as you extend the elbows parallel to the floor. This is *Gassho*.

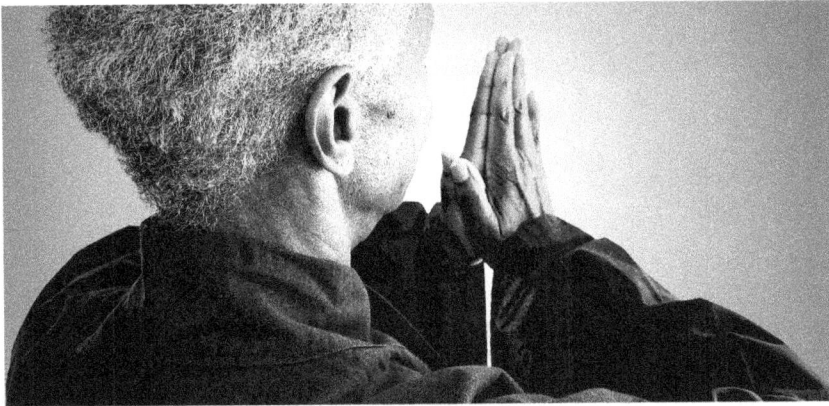

Hands placed in *Gassho*, palms are pressed together, in front and a bit away from the face, and forearms are parallel to the floor (author's collection).

This hand mudra reflects embracing Dharma. It is also a respectful and deeply spiritual part of the importance of forms in Buddhism.

You'll observe *Gassho* when walking past others or when you greet someone. It's also included in bowing by Zen Buddhists and other Buddhists as well.

Even with the release of *Gassho*, Zen Buddhist practitioners have another hand mudra to use when walking around or standing. It's called *Shashu*. To make this mudra, close your fingers around your thumb on your left hand and make a fist. Keep the left fist tight without it being uncomfortable. Now wrap the right fingers just over the knuckles of the left hand while placing the right thumb across the fist-hidden thumb of the left. This is *Shashu*. This mudra is held at your sternum with the elbows extended forming a straight line. *Shashu* is kept while walking or standing, either outside or inside of buildings.

The Cosmic Mudra

Mudras are ways of holding the body that are considered sacred. They also generate energy and can be used therapeutically (Kumar et al., 2018). We have full body mudras and hand mudras. Often you see

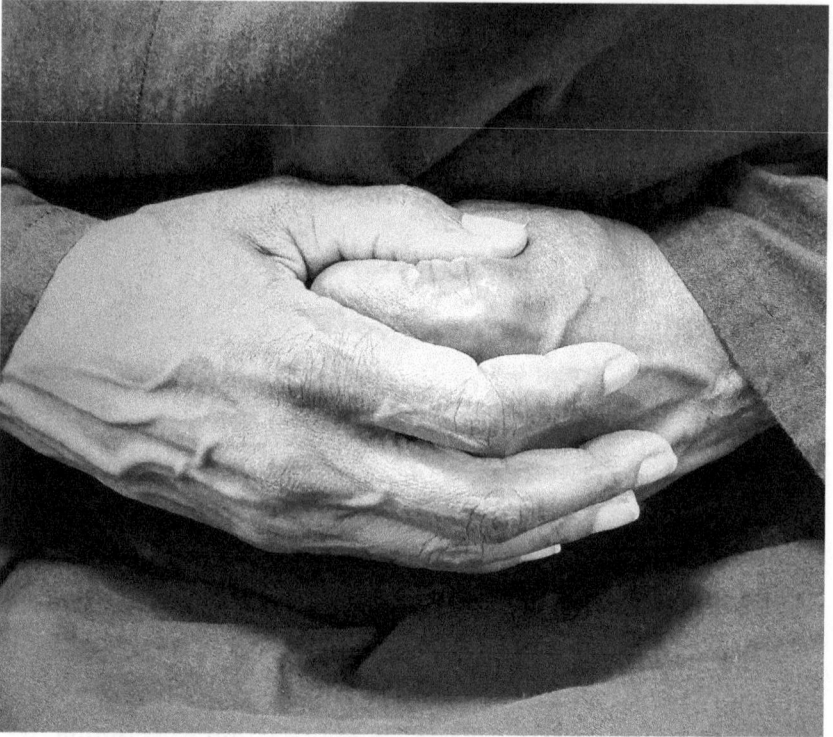

Hands placed in *Shashu*, with the left-hand fingers clasping the left thumb, while the right-hand thumb covers the left and the right-hand fingers wrap around the left-hand fingers (author's collection).

people holding their hands in mudra positions when they meditate. Some have the thumb and middle finger touching. Others sit with the back of their hands with palms upward resting on their legs. For our practice, the mudra generates connection with cosmic forces.

The *Cosmic Mudra* is how we place our hands when doing Zazen. Rest your right hand with the palm up on your lap. Then put your left hand with the palm up on top of the left palm. Next, bring the tips of your two thumbs to just barely touching each other. Now, the placement. Move your *Cosmic Mudra* in front of your navel and your arms slightly away from your body. For Zen Buddhists, this mudra is meant to connect with your *Hara*, or the energy center

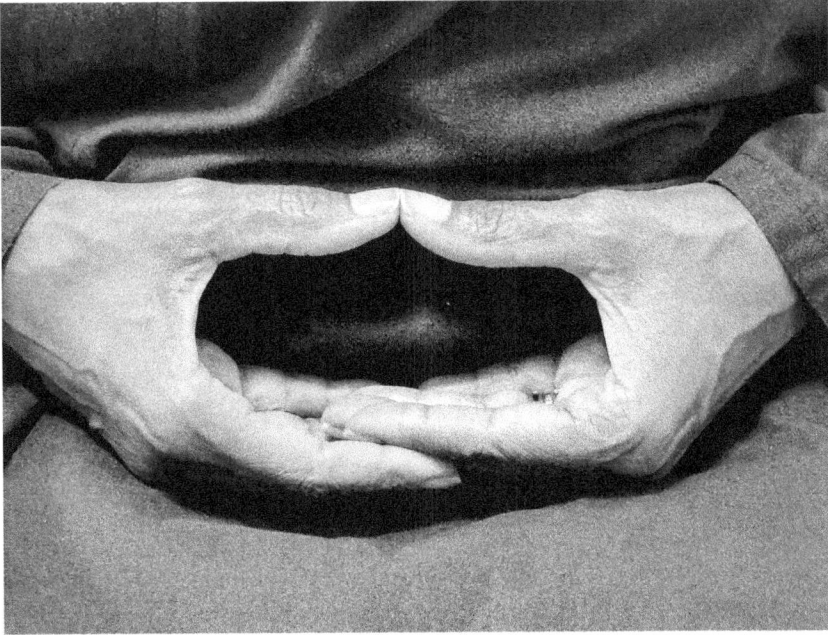

Hands placed in the *Cosmic Mudra*, with the right hand cradling the left hand, while thumbs slightly touch (author's collection).

found in the lower abdomen. Keep your hands "active" as you hold them; feel the energy in them. When doing Zazen we hold our hands in this way. Zazen is itself a full body mudra. It ignites cosmic energy as well as the seeing of your human being without hindrance of your long developed and controlling ego.

Zazen and Kinhin *Meditations*

Zazen is the meditation practice used in Zen Buddhism, as I mentioned earlier. It's "Right Meditation" and also serves as the active and attentive practice point in the *Wisdom Paramita* of concentration. It's a mudra on its own, which encompasses the *Cosmic Mudra.* You'll set up a space where you can face a wall that has nothing on it if you can. We call that facing a blank wall. You can use pillows or cushions to sit on the floor, or a chair, or you can lie down in your bed or on the floor. In a Zazen meditation hall, people have defined things to sit on, like zafus and zabutons. At home, just make sure you have the cushioning you'll need. I'll go over all of this now.

After you find the space you'll use, arrange your cushions so you can be comfortable as you'll sit in an upright position. A zabuton goes on the floor, and a zafu is placed in the center of it. If possible you'll want to sit on the zafu in a Lotus or half Lotus position. That's with the legs crossed and the feet resting on the inner thighs, or one foot resting on the inner thigh. The idea is to use the knees to provide a fulcrum for the hips and upper body. Therefore, you're not sitting flat on the zafu. You are sitting sort of on the edge of it. If you can't do either of those Lotus positions, that's fine, just sit cross-legged like the children do during story time, keeping the leverage over the knees to help the hips and lower back. After you have found a comfortable place for your feet, then you'll sway a little from side to side and back and forth. What you're looking for is feeling your sit bones so that you're not slouching or leaning, supporting your straight spine. Consider your ears; they are positioned over your shoulders so you're pulling in your chin. The top of your head is reaching for the sky. You sit with the eyes open, with your gaze downward at about 45 degrees. Eyes are soft, eyebrows relaxed. So you don't stare directly straight out. Shift your focus so that it's toward the floor. You'll be facing a blank wall, on cushions and pillows if you can, with the hands in the *Cosmic Mudra*. Some people can only sit in a chair. That's fine too, make yourself comfortable and sit upright with the *Cosmic Mudra* and straight spine as I described for sitting on the floor. If you need pillows to support your back and cushion your bottom, and your feet, that's totally all right too. If you can't sit in a chair you may lie on your back. Keep the spine straight, put pillows under your knees, and place your hands in the cosmic mudra. If your back isn't available, you may lay on your right side. In this position, you place your knees as if you were sitting in a chair, then extend the right knee slightly and place your hands with the palms together under your right cheek. (This is hand placement in *Gassho* which I described a few pages ago.). Whatever position works for you, and they can change from day to day or month to month, just sit without reflexively moving. Try to avoid the urge to scratch an itch or wipe a nose tickle or unfurl your legs if they fall asleep, or any other movement. Of course, torture isn't the goal so if you absolutely need to move, please do so. Try sitting still as possible, listen to the silence, and focus on breathing.

The point is that though Zazen appears to be sitting still, it is a movement—a dance meditation actively connecting with cosmic forces and generating energy sitting quietly, sitting in a *mudra* form of Buddha Dharma, and allowing you to forget yourself for a little

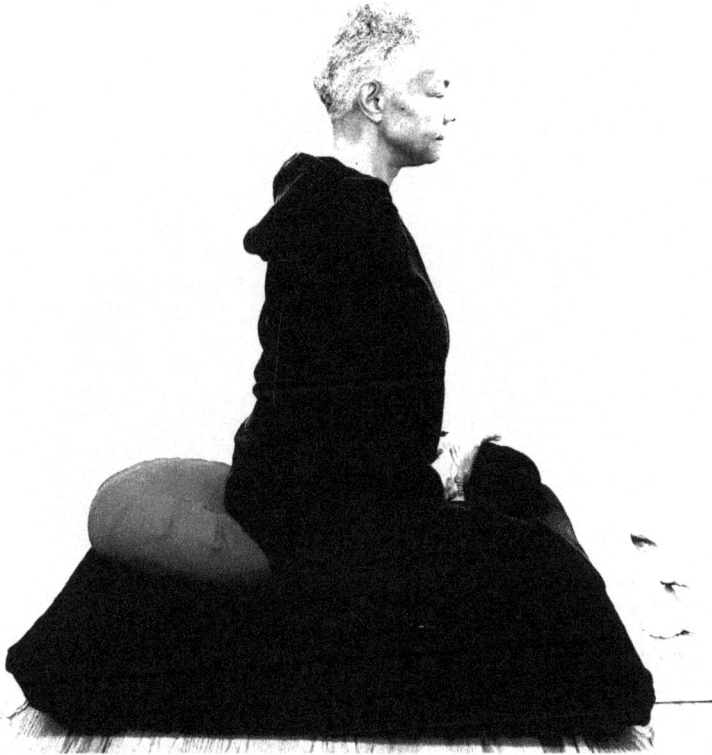

Floor cushion, seated half lotus Zazen posture, with hands in the *Cosmic Mudra*. Spine is erect, head is held with ears aligned with the shoulders, eyes are slightly cast downward (author's collection).

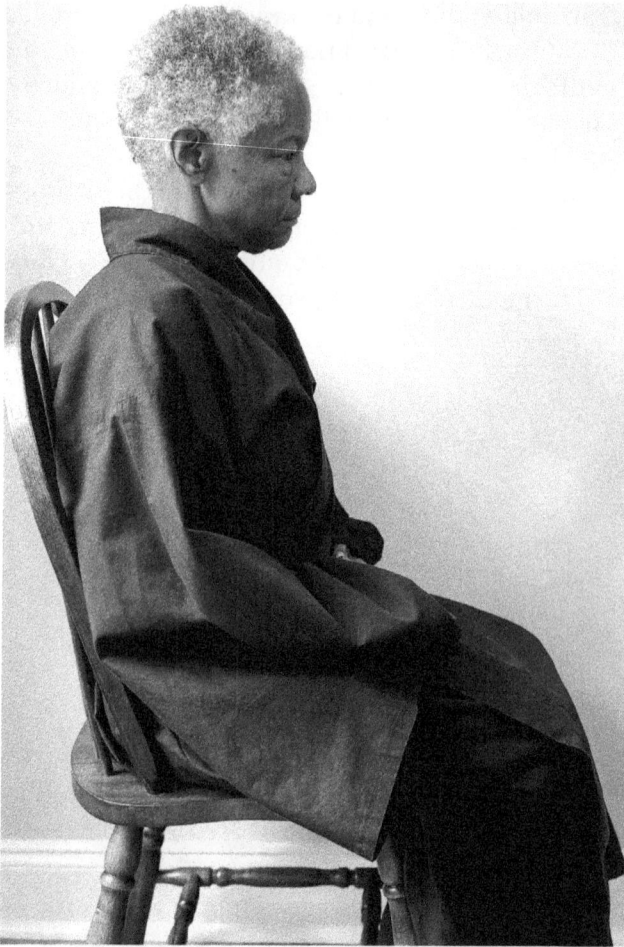

Chair-seated Zazen posture with hands in the *Cosmic Mudra*. Spine is erect, head is held with ears aligned with the shoulders, eyes are slightly cast downward (author's collection).

while. There isn't anything to gain except just sitting being active. You don't slump, do relax your shoulders, and pull your spine upward out of the hips. You don't let your head lean forward or backwards or side to side as you actively pull in your chin. You think about your hands and the energy in the belly, and activate it. Your focus is on your breath, which is what keeps you alive. You notice the silence. Notice the stillness and try to notice it even more as you sit actively.

The goal isn't to stop thinking but to get beyond it just like when you dance. A Dance Dharma while sitting. At first, it's helpful to focus on and count your "inhales" until you get to ten or until you forget what number you're on, in which case you restart each time at one.

Sitting Zazen isn't only for yourself. It is for your family, people you work with, community and the greater world and universe around us. It's a way to be with Sangha, the Buddhists who are on this path as well. In this way when we talk about Right Meditation as part of the Noble Eightfold Path, we are dropping away our egos and realizing we aren't separate from other beings. With practice, you'll find your connection with people changes, your intentions also change, and your mind can rest.

Ordinarily, after a seated Zazen practice with more than one session, we also do walking meditation, or what's called *Kinhin*. Seated Zazen and Kinhin go together. Yes, you can do *Kinhin* as a stand-alone, of course. In practice they are meant to go together. Some have said that walking meditation as we know it is a *Sutra* walk. *Sutras* are the words of Buddhas and Ancestors preserved for us to learn their teachings. That idea can be further simplified for our use, as a *Sutra* is something arising from an Awakened Mind. *Kinhin* is silent Sutra walking, one aspect of Dance Dharma done in the meditation hall or what's often called the *Zendo* that complements Zazen. *Kinhin* is done in different Buddhist practices and it can be done at a fast or slow pace. Some places mix the two. In Zen Buddhism, it's a slow walk. We place attentiveness on being here right now into the body and mind. Feel the floor with your feet, feel the hands, feel the propelling of yourself through space very slowly. Do you notice the space? How's your breath? It's just the same as you inhale and exhale, walking with your gaze out in front of you toward the floor, without bending your neck or tilting your head.

Stand as if you were still in the Zazen sitting position so your back and everything is straight. Put your hands in *Shashu* as I described above, with your right hand clasping your left, the left thumb tucked into the palm of the left hand, the right hand placed around it. For

Kinhin, take the first step with your right foot. Advance by taking only a step for each full breath (one exhalation and inhalation). So, on the first step with the right foot, inhale and exhale slowly. On your next inhale with the left foot, step on the heel, exhale, you exhale before you inhale and step on the right. Keep going. Keep the steps really small. I like to inhale with my right heel, exhale, and simultaneously bring my left heel just to the middle of the right foot and inhale. Then repeat.

Not everyone has Zazen in a *Zendo*. You, like me, may do Zazen at home, or in an office, or outdoors. If you're doing this in a small space, simply make as large a circle as your space allows, going in a clockwise direction. If you have a larger space either indoors or outside, it's up to you. Typically you'll circumambulate the space clockwise as you take your small steps with inhales and exhales. This style of *Kinhin* is a very slow movement meditation lasting about ten minutes. When *Kinhin* is finished, align your feet and do a standing bow, with your hands still held in *Shashu*. If you're with others in a Zen center or monastery, you'll be signaled to start *Kinhin* and end *Kinhin* with bells and clackers. If you're by yourself you can use a mobile app if you like to set up timers and bells for both Zazen and *Kinhin*. Whenever the period of *Kinhin* is finished, after the standing bow, walk quickly back to your sitting cushion. Customarily *Kinhin* is done when there are two or more periods of Zazen going on back to back.

You can think of *Kinhin* as I said, as a mindful dance, as was put by one writer:

> The core essence of Kinhin lies in mindful walking—one step at a time, each infused with [attentiveness]. While walking may seem automatic in our daily lives, approaching it with mindfulness unravels its inherent beauty. Walking slowly, attentively shifting weight from one foot to the other, transforms a seemingly mundane act into a meditative dance. The effects of Kinhin permeate various aspects of life, enhancing sitting meditation, instilling calmness, and fostering mindfulness in routine activities [Swami, 2024; (bracketed change is the author's)].

Kinhin brings us the benefit of getting out of being automatons in our daily lives, I believe this dance can be engaged in between periods of Zazen or on its own. I once taught a class on sacred dance and

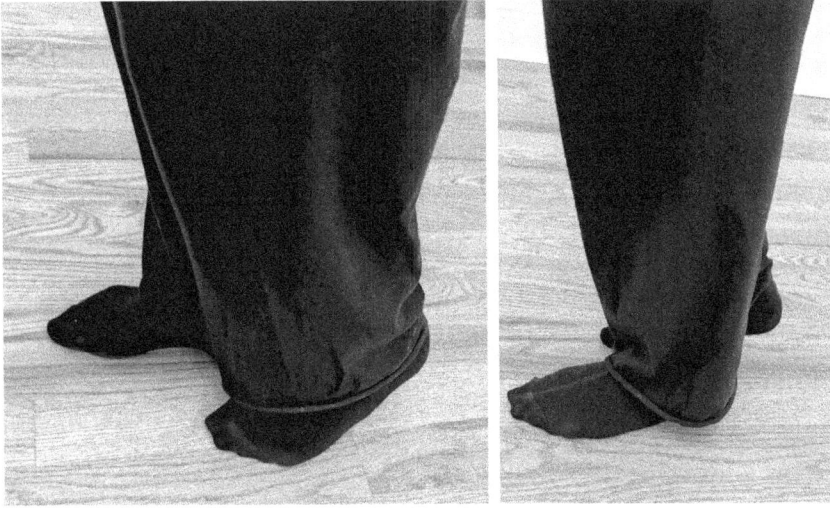

Steps in *Kinhin*, with right foot and then left foot (author's collection).

incorporated *Kinhin* into it. When I asked the undergraduate students what they felt after five minutes of this Dance Dharma, they said they felt calmer and at ease—not so anxious. Like the dance therapy I talked about earlier in this chapter, walking meditation may help with some health issues, such as:

- Cardiotoxicity of anthracycline chemotherapy in people with breast cancer
- Parkinson's disease
- Ankle weakness
- Balance for older people to help reduce falls
- Increase exercise capacity and quality of life
- Glycemic control and vascular function in people with type 2 diabetes
- Depression

So as you dance in *Kinhin*, know that there are very important benefits physically and mentally. Indeed, the Buddhas and Ancestors practiced *Kinhin*. With that having been said, now, let me turn to the Buddha's Awakening.

Part One

Touch Earth

After leaving his family and his very wealthy royal life, a young adult Shakyamuni Buddha came to his enlightenment between 495 and 485 BCE (Mark, 2020). There is a very long history of the Buddha's spiritual path. For now I'm going to start at his awakening. At that point he revealed the *Four Noble Truths* and the *Noble Eightfold Path* as his formula for reducing suffering. He became attentive to these truths as he sat under a Bodhi Tree with his hands in the Cosmic Mudra and practicing the Dance Dharma of Zazen. He also said that he was unaware of these truths and the path before he fully awakened. After he became aware of how to end suffering, that is, letting go of every attachment and self-definition contained in them, he began sharing the Dharma.

Over the course of his remaining life, the Buddha practiced Zazen and shared the Dharma with many assemblies of people. Many Sutras are attributed to the Buddha, and are the bedrock of Buddha Dharma as Zen Buddhists see them.

Importantly, we learn from the Buddha about other buddhas. A buddha is a person, any person, who has completely become attentive to the causes of suffering and the solution to them, who practices Zazen and has an aspiration for enlightenment. It's a person who realizes and opens to his or her vast potential of wisdom. A buddha is one who has brought a final end to suffering and frustration, and knows of happiness and peace based on practice realization.

As long as we hold on to who we think we are, we'll be stuck. Let it all go. That's what Shakyamuni Buddha did. He set aside all that he believed about himself and the world. He evaluated everything he'd been told about who he was and how he was separate from everyone and every being. Along the way he had different starts and stops, with ups and downs. He didn't settle until he realized that it was ego and human beings' ways of putting themselves at the center of the universe that set up causes and conditions that led to suffering. In the spiritual realm too, the Buddha realized he could advocate all day long and for eons for his own singular enlightenment and awareness. Compassionately, he soon realized that it wouldn't do any good if only he were enlightened. Everyone needs to be. What good would it do if he didn't have concern for others?

So he followed the *Four Noble Truths* and the *Noble Eightfold Path*. Took the Buddhist vows and engaged the *Wisdom Paramitas*. After that he proceeded to teach this Dharma. The teachings he gave were oral and have been transcribed and transmitted. The Buddha sat in Zazen and did what I've described as dance meditation *Kinhin* after he was awakened and continued this until the end of his life. While the Buddha was on the earth, he and the others with him did walking meditation, or Dance Dharma, called circumambulation. It was a regular practice after having periods of Zazen, movement in stillness. Before the Buddha received such an honored position, he was a Bodhisattva. This is a person who commits to helping others to realize their true selves.

Bodhisattva Path

In Zen Buddhism and other Buddhist schools, people vow to help others as a way of life. The reason for these vows, expounded first by the Buddha, articulates the truth that if we don't help others we aren't helping ourselves. When the focus is only on securing *my* salvation, *my* healing, *my* joy, it leaves so many people out. It's an ego-focused spiritual pride in a way, with "self" doing all the driving.

Like Shakyamuni Buddha, we recognize that all beings we encounter suffer, regardless of their position at the time we interact with them. And all things are impermanent, which in itself gives us the feeling of suffering. A Bodhisattva recognizes this and instead of focusing on their selves, turns the focus to helping others. This isn't an addictive kind of overstepping of boundaries mind you. It is rather a shift in the mental perception of "me first, you second" or "I'm not you" or "You are separate from me" in everything, every action. The Bodhisattva point of view is filled with compassion and wisdom as they take beneficial and identity action, speak kindly, and make giving their main way of being. Each thought or action or intention is imbued with *Wisdom Paramitas* and the vows they've taken, as

I pointed out earlier. Rather than being driven by greed, anger and hate, or delusion, they are activated by the promise to help all beings see their true selves. This is the heart of the Buddha's teaching, which he instilled from his own experience. From that experience, we learn through *Sutras* and Dharma teachers that a Bodhisattva has also agreed to help beings transition from the cycle of life and death.

What Is Birth and Death? A Change in Form

Earlier in the book, I talked about my childhood death experiences, and exposure early on to the fact and feeling of impermanence. At the time, I had no particular concepts of death that I was aware of. It was like I had no need to grieve, though I did feel my father's absence. He didn't come home anymore. I didn't know what it meant that he died. I knew there was a vacancy, a void where he once was, even though he caused lots of suffering for me and my mother and sisters and his loved ones and family.

And no one talked about death either. No one said, hey, he's in a better place, or he's probably in heaven, or he deserved to go to hell. These statements are like those that I've heard over the years when someone dies. Admittedly, there were no conversations, no explanations, no idea of grief counseling or groups—just a deep and long-lasting sad, silent, regretful void, left over remembrance of that person's consciousness, where violence used to prevail and now it didn't. I didn't begin to feel sad, I'm now concluding, as at the time, I didn't have any attachment to the concepts of loss of a loved one through death.

The churches that I would attend much later were versed in heaven and hell, and none of them agreed on how, when, and how long one would stay in hell, or when "resurrection" or "rapture" would occur. People held on to their loved ones and wanted them to stay "on this side" no matter how badly they were suffering, for example, in the hospital with comas and intubations. And there are movies and programs that dramatize death and the sadness that comes from losing someone to it.

For me, I'm not saying losing a loved one is a happy time. It isn't usually. We miss them, we want to talk with them, maybe apologize for something, or try harder to have a relationship with them. What is true I think is that people are scared of dying on some level at some point, which is learned. This is evident knowing it's not clear exactly the destination at death of the so-called breath and mind that animated the body. This actually is the entire reason for many people's religious practices: to know why we're here and what happens to us after we die.

The reason I appreciate the Zen Buddhist approach to that question is it doesn't claim to know, to have any answers. What it does claim is that the body is made of the earthly elements, air, water, fire, and earth. That we break down into matter, alive or dead, and as we know from Einstein, matter is neither created nor destroyed. And the Buddha explained the teaching of emptiness, that is, we do not have anything that we can hold onto: We and everything in our constructed world are impermanent and depend in some way on others. At the point of death, when the breath ceases and mind stops, our bodies are transformed like a piece of wood in a fireplace. We are changed from one form to another. I noted this to be the case with my father. He as a body was no longer there, his void was, and for many of those in my family, it still is. We know him as his form that has been abandoned.

This sort of approach to just being with death can be a bit tricky for people who have a strong belief in heaven and hell dualities, and maybe reincarnation, which I'll talk about in a moment. Simply, these life and death points of view serve as concepts to explain the main question. Perhaps these are dualistic ideas to help us deal with the fact of impermanence, to help us feel like we have some control over life. Now I know there are theories of "out of body" death experiences too. We hear from people what they saw when they were unconscious. It's fine for me to hold the birth and death cycle loosely so that everyone can do an inquiry into it for themselves without relying on dualistic thinking.

Cause and Effect

When people die, some believe that they come back to live in different reincarnate bodies with the same consciousness. And they come back to live in this way due to karma, or cause and effect. You've heard it: You reap what you sow. And, of course we know that with each movement, motion, push, intention, physical, mental thought or emotion, there is a result. Infrequently it appears with immediate visibility and on occasion it seems to appear later without our knowing. And this kind of approach to existence of beings peppers many Buddhist traditions.

Zen Buddhism, though, suggests causes and conditions produce effects, and rebirths. These effects are stored in our minds, our consciouses. They originate with everything and everyone else, called *co-origination* or *dependent origination*.

Co-origination means "if this, then that." It means nothing arises without others, whether sentient or insentient. It means we can't create ourselves or live without others. Trying to do each of the steps required to feed yourself, for example, growing the food or making your way to fix an air conditioner on the fritz, can't be done without the help of others. *Co-origination* takes the idea of rebirth and puts it on a cycle to show that birth of suffering comes from ignorance, and that in turn produces an unskillful action that we think will somehow relieve the suffering, only it leads to more suffering, and so we give rise to birthing more suffering. At its heart, the seeking for good feelings to relieve suffering comes from the deep-seated need for love and affection. In our ignorance we seek unwholesome things: buying stuff, sexual stuff, food stuff, and so on. It doesn't ever fill that need so we keep on trying and stay on this wheel of suffering. That's cause and effect, and at the same time *co-origination*.

Some have suggested that the idea of rebirth and reincarnation is also a linked chain of causation, which makes people seek out a new body or makes people accept a new body at death, depending on how they behaved in the last life. What I know today is that each one of us has to take the time to consider these ideas. At the same time, we should study what we know about birth and death, and consider what we believe and why. It's important to loosen the grasp we have on what we have been conditioned to be the truth of birth, death, heaven, hell, and everything in between. Approaching everything from the perspective of the *Noble Eightfold Path* and within the fluid rings of the *Wisdom Paramitas* and the Precepts helps us release and find the fundamental point of living here on Earth.[2] The Buddha purposely left aside providing specific answers to elusive questions on death. Instead the notion that life and death go together were his stance, and this stance has come to us through Zen Buddhist practice. Coming to this understanding is one aspect of enlightenment.

Enlightenment

In the last pages, I've given an overview of Dance Dharma. And in them, I've attempted to explain how walking meditation, or *Kinhin*, is a Dance Dharma. At the same time, I've broached the point that Zazen is an active movement, not a stagnant kind of practice, and it's one kind of Dance Dharma. When we sit we also dance. It's nice also to note that Dance Dharma is nondiscursive, nonverbal, and nondual. Dharma in terms of Zen Buddhism originates with the Buddha. Dharma with a capital D means his true teachings, which are called the Treasury of the True Dharma Eye, or a jewel, or a wonderful opportunity by the Ancestors. Through our Zen practice, we can see more clearly with it. We can become what's called enlightened. Zen Buddhism enlightenment can be had in an instant, and repeatedly or along a gradual line that spirals up and down. The main point is that *enlightenment* isn't a destination. Enlightenment is now, it's realizing your practice of Zazen and appreciating your life in totality. You understand that just this is it. Attentiveness to each and every moment, all the ups and downs, every afront to your ego is a request to realize how you're conditioned and constructed in such a way that you'll just keep being blind to your Way Seeking Mind, your call to become a Bodhisattva and help everyone. Instead of just reacting to each situation, you become able to render an appropriate response.

Listen, I'm not saying sainthood is what this is, or rigidness is required. It's certainly not. What I'm saying is the realization of impermanence and the focus on knowing you're not separate from any being, that you have mountains, rivers, city streets or country roads to cross, poor treatment of our fellows in and outside of our ethnic identities, work, family, and all the accoutrements of being human to deal with. And let's not forget antiblack racism or sexism or any of the other ills that people suffer from as a result of greed, hate and anger, and delusion. There's no running away; there is no place to go. Even your garbage and sewage wind up somewhere on this earth.

Zen Buddhist practices acknowledge and embrace life and everything it brings, including death, welcomes it all in. The teachings say each and every thing or event is likely a manifestation of the Buddha, asking you, guiding you, through gates unknown to you leading to enlightenment. Once you have it, you must keep it well.[3] Pursuit of anything no matter how large or small can be delusional, and nothing is ever as it seems. Accepting this and working with the reality of it with a skillful response is enlightenment. To move and dance forward with this kind of enlightenment means practice. It's not a one-time thing. We have to establish a routine for practice, just like we vow to do to end suffering.

Establish Daily Practice

Daily practice of Zazen is very important to realizing that you have enlightenment and it occurs right here in your daily life, with all the struggles and joys. Having a daily practice also means remembering that there is birth embedded in death too. In sitting Zazen every day, we have the chance to look at our egos and understand our consciousnesses. Let go of greed, anger and hate, and at least recognize delusion. We deepen our compassion for everyone. We acknowledge that we aren't sitting in meditation in the mindfulness market. We sit Zazen meditation for others on this crazy planet. We want to help other people and ourselves get better, and come to practice realization for themselves. Develop the "Way Seeking Mind" (Sunryu, 2011). We therefore sit Zazen not expecting to gain a single thing.

As I said earlier, you'll need a spot where you can place a cushion or chair, or a space to lie down on if you can't sit, and face a wall that isn't cluttered. You may benefit from a timer, either on your phone or otherwise, without giving in to the urge to constantly check the time. Set a timer depending on your experience. Some people who are brand new to sitting start with just a few minutes and increase the time gradually over weeks and months. The point is to sit every day and if you can, at the same time each day in the same location. A lot of us get up early before everyone else, especially if there are people living with or near you who aren't with you on the path.

You'll want to find other people to practice with too. That's your Sangha. You support them and they support you. Some places have Zazen in the morning, evening during the week, and have opportunities on the weekends. Lots of Zen centers offer online Zazen. I've put a few of these in the Places to Practice section of this book. You can also do a search online to see what centers are near you. They're all over the place in the United States and in different countries. You'll get many different results. As you'll try different places some will resonate, some won't. You might find you like several of them. Please give each place you try a few chances. Talk to the teachers you find there. Nearly all people are a bit shy when they start out, worried they'll make a mistake or something. Just let those doubts go. One thing about getting connected with a Sangha is the awesome aspect of finding a teacher, an authentically transmitted teacher.

Why a Teacher Is Important

Yes, there are Zen Buddhist and other Buddhist teachers. It's important that you find one to work with and one that practices with the True Dharma Eye. I'm a Soto Zen Buddhist under the Suzuki Roshi lineage out of San Francisco Zen Center in California. Other Soto Zen lineages have subtle differences from the lineage I belong to. Like anything, you have to investigate and engage until you feel comfortable, and find someone you can stick with.

Many teachers will work with you via Zoom if needed if you aren't in close physical proximity. Working with a teacher, it's not like you might think. A good teacher is hard to find, they say—it's a person you can talk to, can share with, practice with, who won't exactly tell you what to do as they guide your practice. They don't have to be like you in gender or age or skin color. They just have to be fully committed to the authentic Buddha Dharma, and have had ordination. That generally means they will have a title of Zen Priest. Despite designations, there are many levels of teachers and no two are the same in their manor or method.

This has been a long winding chapter, giving you the vision of dance as Dharma, the rituals of bowing, the mudras of Zazen. I've provided a short overview of the Buddha's enlightenment, and talked generally about being a Bodhisattva. Life and death, cause and effect, and what that means in this practice were talked about just for a moment or two. And then, I broached the topic of enlightenment, particularly explaining it's not a destination. It's a ride. Practice enlightenment involves Zazen and daily practice, and working with a teacher. And these are the practices that sustain our lives, no matter what. From here, I'll turn to the using the practices of Dance Dharma and Zazen to help support cancer treatment, and provide some idea of the landscape of health care for American Blacks and other people who have experienced racism.

Part Two

Dance Dharma, Zazen, and Multiple Myeloma

My Journey

Medicine and disease subdue each other. What is yourself?
—Ch'ung-hsien, 2006, p. 382

The Diagnosis

Dancing had always benefited me. As a young girl, I checked books out of the library on ballet and practiced the positions. When I was in junior high, I chose dance and gymnastics instead of general physical exercise, or PE (physical education) class since I loved dance in the way it allowed "dropping away of body and mind," as I'd eventually learn it was called in Zen Buddhism. This *Dance Dharma* meant being freed from attachments weighing me down and stressing me out.

With my belief in the power of dance, I started a dance company. My private dance company attracted students of all ages and ethnicities. I taught ballet for beginners and advanced dancers, and choreographed performances. At the same time, I taught a special type of dance, sacred dance meditation, which drew on First Nation practices from before the Common Era. Those people knew and embodied connections from all sorts of energies and spiritual realms. Shamans, kamis, stupas, star gods, Medicine Wheels: All kinds of methods mitigating negative energies and upholding positive ones were known and venerated. These were there and accessible for the well-being of all. So, I danced and drew in these energies and shared them with interested people.

Part Two

As of then, I had never had any type of chronic or acute illness or disease. With my race and ethnicities, I knew that certain chronic diseases—comorbidities as they're called—such as diabetes, hypertension, and cholesterol-related issues were expected to make my life difficult. They would also doom me to taking daily prescriptions, and eventually, end my life early.

At any rate, comorbidities weren't my history at all. I grew up in poverty and my family wasn't able to get good medical care. I remember how my mother used to get really angry when one of us three girls got sick or broke a bone or something at school or outside playing. And my parents hardly ever went to the doctor. The dentist? No, a dentist was visited only when it was too late to save a tooth or there was an emergency. I didn't start regular dental care until I was able to cover the costs myself.

Anyway, through my education and my career I'd learned about diseases that seem prevalent among American Black and poor people, and what to do to avoid them, such as eating right and exercising, getting enough rest and relaxation, staying hydrated, and the importance of regular dental care. I practiced all of these, and also abstained from any and all intoxicants, didn't smoke, and visited the general medical practitioner each year. Over time, I established quarterly visits to the dentist and later added the periodontist, for cleanings, since there is a connection between periodontal disease and cancers, diabetes, hypertension, and kidney problems (Chatzopoulos et al., 2024). From time to time I had a behavioral therapist too, even though my family and the then current culture were like many who scoffed at using that kind of support. "Why should I go there and tell all my business? I'm doing fine just as I am," they'd say as they maybe lit a cigarette or drank some liquor, or other escape.

One day I was minding my own business, teaching dance, choreographing, and just being with my life. My general practice doctor (GP from now on), who I searched for, interviewed, and began seeing a couple of years earlier, called to say my blood tests needed to be redone. He said there was a technical error with the phlebotomist. They'd done the tests the prior month, in November when I went in for my annual checkup. So I went back in, just after Thanksgiving. They drew my blood and said they'd be in touch.

Early in December I was participating a seven-day silent retreat called a *Rohatsu* Sesshin at San Francisco Zen Center. It's an annual period of time when Buddhists celebrate Buddha's Enlightenment by sitting Zazen. I was lying in bed on a short break. My phone buzzed. The caller ID "Hematology Oncology" traveled across the screen. You're not supposed to talk during sesshin. Pushing through a little guilt, I answered this one.

"Hi this is Courtenay at the hematology oncology office, calling to schedule your appointment. Your GP referred you."

"What? He didn't tell me anything about this. What's this for?"

She said the same thing she already said, and added, "We can get you in tomorrow. Your GP wanted you to be seen immediately."

I said the same thing I already said, and then, "No, let me call you back."

"Okay, but you need to be seen right away, and since you have a referral marked urgent, I can get you scheduled pretty quick."

All I managed was a bewildered, "Thank you."

When I got to the airport on my way back home, I called my GP. Naturally I had to leave a message. When he called me back, I asked him, after the niceties, "Why have you referred me to a hematology oncologist?"

"Your blood proteins are abnormally high, and that's why we wanted to double check your blood work last month. The second set of labs showed your immunoglobulins and blood protein levels were even higher than they were with the first test."

"Why didn't you call me and let me know, rather than just have an oncologist call me out of the blue? What do my lab results mean?"

"I think you should go to the oncologist and talk to him. He's an expert and can explain it to you better than I can."

He never gave me a straight answer, only just kept saying the same words. Now, I had a great deal of respect for the GP, since he was an osteopathic practitioner with an MD degree. I'd been going to him for a couple of years. This GP relied more on the body's healing

abilities, lifestyle, and diet support for living well, and less on quick fixes with big pharma.

About six weeks later, I went in to see the oncologist only since I was getting progressively worse. I couldn't dance, my back was hurting, and no chiropractic or massage therapy was helping. My weight was dropping like an airplane out of fuel.

The oncologist, Dr. W., introduced himself, then asked in his Italian accent, "Do you know what you have?"

He was short, with black curly hair and olive toned skin. He didn't wear a white coat, and was jacketless with a long sleeved light blue shirt and tie. His male nurse practitioner, blond, who towered over him, stood behind him in his white coat, tapping with one hand on a laptop he held in other hand. I assumed he was writing notes on the conversation, even as he never looked up.

"Multiple myeloma?" I answered, feeling really irritated. Why was he asking me and not telling me? Yes, I had done a bit of research on all my symptoms, which clearly pointed to the disease. I was terrified and scared. All I'd uncovered was the certain fatality I faced from this rare and deadly blood cancer that eats bones like termites eat wood, taking over my bone marrow.

His affirmation of my own diagnosis followed: "With your genetic risk factors and off the charts high levels of immunoglobulins, you'll die soon without treatment, and you'll probably live only a few years in any event. The cancer isn't curable," he said, "but your life can be extended with chemotherapy infusions, followed by an autologous bone marrow transplant and, after that, maintenance with monoclonal antibodies. The disease is terminal though, and eventually you'll be overtaken by it or by infections your immune system can't mitigate. I want you to go see my colleague too, he's a specialist in these matters."

The exam room spun as he spoke. Standing, which I'd been doing since I arrived, I steadied myself by reaching out for the wall. And I turned to look at it.

"Please have a seat," he gestured toward the chair next to the one my husband sat in.

"It's too painful, I'd rather stand." I kept looking at the wall and felt the anger, confusion, the "I can't believe this?" welling up. He's got to be kidding me.

"Do you want some oxycodone for the pain? I can give you some now and also call in prescription. Or do you want something stronger?" He raised his eyebrows.

"No, thank you." I shook my head, exhaled. I tried to focus on my *hara* and my breath. I glanced at my husband, sitting slightly behind me. He got up and put his hand on my shoulder.

The doctor continued, "Please start taking the blood thinner to avoid strokes, which this disease causes, by the way, by thickening your blood, and take the antiviral too so you won't get shingles or other viruses. Your immune system is totally compromised. Antiviral meds will help protect it. I've called these into your pharmacy along with the oxycodone. After you finish the tests I've ordered, please come and see me. My scheduler will set it up. If you have any questions, just give us a call. If you have any problems with stroke or heart attack, go to the emergency room, I'm on staff at Piedmont."

"Is this a disease mainly affecting Black people? I read that it was."

He crossed his arms. "We don't care if you're Black, I'm from Italy and this doesn't matter to me." He looked from me to my white husband and back.

We left like two sheep lost from a herd, with a stack of emergency medical orders for bone marrow biopsy, full body MRI, urine flow test, kidney function test, and CT scan, echocardiogram, and prescriptions, one for oral chemo, one for antiviral meds, one for anticoagulant, and more than eight others for all the side effects associated with them. The tests were to confirm my diagnosis, which they did, and it was forever set in stone on my medical chart within the next three weeks: MM, high risk, spine fractures, not in remission, female at birth, Black, Buddhist.

I cried all the time.

A couple of weeks after this, I'd planned to go to a Mountain Seat Ceremony honoring my teacher's newly appointed position as Abbot of Green Dragon Temple Monastery, part of the San Francisco Zen Center, and then to another sesshin in April. April sesshins commemorate Buddha's birthday. All the arrangements were set, including my airline tickets from Atlanta to San Francisco. My practice led me to the monastery where my teacher was and we met somewhat regularly while I lived in California, and more regularly after the pandemic on Zoom, and when I moved to Georgia.

I emailed him to let him know I wasn't going to make the ceremony or the sesshin. And then we talked. He said he wanted me to let the Sangha, or the Zen community, know I was sick. I didn't want to. I was ashamed and scared and didn't want to connect. And what if the disease went away? Then it would be all the angst for nothing. And besides, I didn't want to bother anyone. After we talked more about this and Well Being Ceremonies, when the community would hold me in their thoughts, he said they should know, they care about you. I said okay. From that point on I was put on Well Being Ceremony lists all over the place, at different temples around the country.

In my little town where I was living, my husband started telling everyone, against my will, about my cancer. Then immediately I was on prayer lists around town. And no, I just wanted to keep it to myself. When people said they'd pray for me, I thought, "Whatever. I wish my husband would stop telling everyone." He didn't.

The Disease of Multiple Myeloma

Everyday fatigue and pain overwhelmed me. For a few minutes each day—for times that were supposed to be breakfast, lunch, and dinner—I'd get out of bed, and without having sat there for more than five minutes, return to lying down in bed, on the living room couch, on the screen porch chaise lounge. When I lay down, my thoughts nearly drove me crazy. *How in the world is this happening to me? What did I do wrong?* No answer came. I thought about all the people I'd known in my life and about how I'd helped or maybe hurt them. All the wrong or poor choices I'd made. *How did I wind up like this after a lifetime of what I thought was intending the best for myself and others?*

This is a sneaky and likely a silent cancer. Lots of people have never heard of it. Those who have it often don't realize it. The disease can smolder for years before any symptoms appear. There can be no symptoms until it's too late often times. People discover they have MM incidentally, like during a routine physical when blood is tested, as in my case. Or when they go to the doctor with an unrelenting backache or a hip and leg ache. Once diagnosed as advanced, personal agency is lost.

Three weeks after the confirmed diagnosis in March, when I could barely walk, bend, or twist my back, sit up in bed, eat or do anything, from the debilitating effects and pain, I was buried under an avalanche of sadness and fear. At the first infusion treatment for chemotherapy, upon taking my medical history, they were curious about why I didn't have comorbidities. The professionals that treated me weren't American Black, except for one nurse. My responses to the medical history questions and their reactions—wow, really? they said—and quizzical facial expressions signaled that I didn't represent the caricature they'd expected from a woman with my skin color in the United States.

When doctors asked if I wanted pain medicines, either for the disease itself or the pain caused by side effects from chemo medications for treating it, I declined, as they went ahead and prescribed them anyway, saying I could pick them up at the pharmacy if I needed them. I tried to explain that rather, for the pain, I would prefer to know what's causing it, treat it, than mask it with pain killers. And I offered that if the pain didn't subside on its own within more than a day, I'd take Tylenol or Advil and lay down. Since I was a dancer all of my life, raising my son alone, in addition to having demanding careers in higher education and municipal finance where stopping and resting weren't actually options, I'd developed a very high pain threshold. If I was performing on stage, and I'd twisted my ankle let's say, I'd take Advil and apply serious amounts of ice, put on an ankle brace, and keep going. And being in leadership at work, I couldn't just not go in each time I had a headache, which was often by the way.

Not too long after being on the daily oral chemo, and just finishing the infusion chemotherapy, I scheduled a visit with a palliative physician for acute pain in my chest and rib area, and multiple "mini strokes." After discussing the situation with her, she wanted to know if I was being honest about not taking pain medicines.

Disbelieving my answer, she asked, "Would you consent to a drug screening right now?"

I felt totally insulted! "Yes, of course that's fine," I said.

The drug test screened for everything from Advil to Xanax. The results were negative for any and all, no over-the-counter analgesics, no prescribed pain or tranquilizer medicines, no CBDs, or street drugs, no nothing.

At the beginning of treatment, lying there at the infusion center or at home, my mind was in a fog, my digestive system wasn't working, I could barely stand or walk, I was dizzy, had excruciating headaches, and I couldn't sit up for long. Standing up required that I let out a vibratory holler from the depths of my *hara* from the pain, and I needed to hold on to the dresser at home to finish the standing, or the chair at the infusion center. I could not simply lie down either. That required that I edge my way onto the bed or examination table and have someone hold my back and arms so they could lean me back onto my left side. I could not roll on to my stomach or lie flat or get to my right side. This all meant that Zazen was difficult to do. Even as that was true, when I lay down, I tried to focus on my breath, and put my hands in the *Cosmic Mudra* as best I could.

It was nearly impossible to do any personal grooming. I had no appetite and was dropping two or three pounds a week even while embarking on the first phase of the three-phased standard of care (SOC) protocol for newly diagnosed MM: proteasome inhibitors (PIs), immunomodulatory drugs (IMiDs), frontline autologous stem cell transplant (ASCT), and anti–CD38 monoclonal antibodies (mABs) (Mateos et al., 2022). The oncologist prescribed the SOC for MM, and drugs that offset the side effects of the treatment—nausea, constipation, headaches, muscle cramps, etc. Of the offsetting drugs prescribed, I refused or stopped taking after trying them. These ancillary medicines caused more problems for me than those that treated the cancer—like nausea, muscle cramps, dizziness, constipation, fatigue, appetite reduction, drowsiness. Here, like before, I also declined all the prescribed and over the counter pain killers. I did take the constipation, anticoagulant, and antiviral prescriptions.

There were so many things I couldn't do that I used to, including intimacy with my husband, vacuuming, watering plants, or taking a hot bath. Not only that, each day I thought about my life with dance being over, like my life had no meaning if I couldn't dance.

Cancer Treatment

After all the emergency screening tests were done, I went back to the Italian oncologist my GP referred me to. My intuition told me I should find someone else, at least see about going to a world class renown cancer center. After checking out several of them around the southeastern United States, I self-referred to the nearest one in Atlanta. I got an appointment within three weeks. I let the Italian oncologist know what my plans were; he called and told my selected oncologist, Dr. C, that they can't wait three weeks to see me, saying that the tumors on my spine and my test results, my advanced stage of cancer, put me close to death within days. So, I got in right away, starting with a video call with the hematology oncology specialist, Dr. C. He was definitely not a person of color! He talked to me about my prognosis sort of, then, within two days, at the beginning of April, I was scheduled for weekly infusion chemotherapy for the next 12 weeks. He prescribed oral chemo meds as well, that I was to take every day for 21 days, then stay off for seven days. It was a two hour drive each way. For me, it was important that I receive the best care without having to fly somewhere to get it. My husband and I braced ourselves for driving, figuring, what the heck, we had long survived LA traffic!

The oncology nurses at the infusion center were knowledgeable and caring, gentle, and supportive. Really all except two were this way, and since I didn't want to deal with those two, I asked that others be my nurses. Those other two were abrupt and "doing their job," so to speak, and being helpful and caring wasn't in their interpretation of their job description. They used needles for inserting the IV device that were too big, couldn't find my veins and wouldn't ask for help (though I have "good veins" which are easy to find). When I said, Could you use a smaller needle?, to one of the nurses, she said they didn't have any of the smaller ones. I knew that wasn't right, they were in plain view in the drawer. When I said, Let's call someone to help you? to the other nurse who was difficult, she said she treats me just like anybody else. I didn't ask her, as I wondered if she thought I was accusing her, that she was treating me different based on my skin color?

Dr. C, at our first in-person visit while discussing the possibilities of an autologous bone marrow transplant, which was by the way the first in-person visit a couple of months into the chemotherapy infusion treatments, responded to my husband's question about whether MM affects more Blacks than whites. He said, no, the people in the medical system treat Blacks as inferior so they get worse care (Geiger, 2003; Derman et al., 2020; Cho et al., 2021). I did learn from searching online that American Blacks and people of color are many more times as likely than whites to get the disease and die more frequently (Kanapuru, 2022).

By comparison, the nurse practitioners came across to me as authoritarians, and questions I had about rashes, or fevers, or mini strokes were answered with a blame the victim tone, with no consideration for maybe understanding or considering my difficulties as being related to the MM chemotherapy medicines. When they needed to examine me for a set of raised hives on my back I told them about, for example, the nurse practitioner was rough: jacking up my clothes without asking me if it was okay, or letting me know she wanted to do that, or asking me and giving me time to adjust to what she wanted. And upon the curt examination conclusion, she said she didn't know what the hives were from. The only thing she said was I could go to the ER if it persists or happens again. Worse, she never said to me that they were a possible side effect of the oral chemo drugs, which should be taken into consideration when assessing dosage (Imbesi et al., 2015; Perez-Kempner, 2019). After reading and researching the possibility of the medication being the cause, I stopped taking it until the hives cleared up.

---

4. Dance Dharma, Zazen, and Multiple Myeloma

While the nurse practitioners were rough on my body, the oncologist never touched me for examinations, didn't use a stethoscope to listen to anything, didn't peer into my eyes or ears, throat, or mouth. He stuck to reading the test results only. And, in reflecting, it was interesting that neither the oncologist or anyone of the care team members told me what to expect from treatment in terms of pain, quality of life, or side effects. When, after the first and second infusion, I had fever and vomiting, I was told to go the emergency room or come to the cancer care center, hours from my house. At least that was what I was told before letting them know I was not going to engage in ASCT (autologous stem cell transpant) as my being high risk made the procedure more dangerous. Here's why:

> For patients of any age who were classified as ... high risk, we report high rates of early mortality and a poor statistical cure fraction, and have not been able to demonstrate a significant improvement in outcome since the early 1990s [with ASCT]. Consequently, improving both short-term and long-term survival in patients with high-risk disease should be a priority for future research [Nishimura et al., 2020, p. 437].

What was my high risk? Genetic factors for one thing, and the level and type of immunoglobulins for another. Genetic factors meant my DNA had been transposed, and the immunoglobulins were so high they were unreadable. And I had tumors on the exterior of my spine, called extramedullary, which mean the cancer was able to reach other organs. A bone marrow transplant would have caused other life-threatening issues as I understood it. And it would have required that I be debilitated for a year, and that my life expectancy would only increase by the same amount. So it was a zero-sum total for me.

It appeared to me that the care actually further declined after I informed the team that I wasn't participating in the transplant protocol. I think that was a revenue-based behavior, coming from the fact that they weren't going to be able to bill me for it. At one point when it was time for the mABs, having opted out of the ASCT, I had to ask if I might get information on how the medicine causes pain or other changes in the body, like risk for stroke or heart attack. In response, the pharmacist on the care team called me and discussed the document she'd sent just before the call, saying there were no side effects from the mABs injections. With one exception, from appearances, the doctors and nurses weren't American Blacks. The medical assistants and the receptionists were. The patients I saw didn't appear to be either.

Patients lay prone or leaned back in their reclining chairs, not moving unless they had to go to the restroom, dragging their IV machine with them like robotic dance partners, as the intravenous fluids kept flowing. The only movement in the infusion room was nurses wheeling around their state-of-the-art computers, blood pressure monitors, and IV bag racks grating on the floor as they rolled. Caregivers accompanying the patients sat still reading their phones and made no noise; went and got something to eat, came back, sat, worried. It's the cultural norm for patients to be still and be quiet, to accept what the SOC dictates, as it was fed to the nurses reading patient's electronic medical charts. Occasionally a question is asked by a patient or caregiver, and always these were done in whispered tones. Snacks and "warm blankets" were provided, especially at the onset of chemotherapy treatment, along with the offering of something to drink. An American Black male volunteer went around to the zombie patients like me that were bound to stillness and passivity, encouraged us by telling stories about his last vacation to Puerto Rico. Honestly at the time, I didn't want to hear about it. I thought there's no way I'll be able to travel anywhere other than this godforsaken place with its mandatory do this treatment. My assumption was that I was going to die way before any vacation could happen and so why waste my time thinking about that. I know he was trying to distract and provide a positive outlook, which is definitely something people under these conditions might benefit from.

Infusion Treatment Progress

The treatment did its job, normalizing my blood protein and immunoglobulins. The DNA was forever mutated and that was that. At the time I was still losing weight, unable to muster any enthusiasm to do anything, and dying inside from depression. Don't lift anything over ten pounds, don't bend or twist your spine, I was told. If you feel sick, go to the ER, surely do continue on all your meds. The social worker I was assigned, after I asked for help, provided a referral to a therapist, who was very helpful. She had no experience with my disease, though she was an American Black woman living in my state. We did telemedicine and that was great. The drugs produced brain fog and fatigue, so that I couldn't remember what I wanted to say, and in my case not being able to move made life feel futile. With all that, I did sit at the computer and interact with her.

Also, the oral chemo medication caused my ribs, spine, and chest to ache to the point where I couldn't turn around to look over my shoulder or bend over to tie my shoes. I discovered that that was caused by the oral chemo when I was off the oral treatment for the required seven days and the pain subsided. I'd previously asked Dr. C to reduce my dose and he'd refused. Later, maybe about three weeks, when I told them that I believed the current dosage was causing neurotoxicity, he agreed to reduce the dosage.

And the oral chemo meds were very expensive, regardless of the dosage. I could only get them from a "specialty pharmacy." I was grateful for health insurance—I would not be able to pay for them otherwise. When I decided I didn't want to renew, as the reduced dosage was still causing pain, the specialty pharmacy kept calling, emailing, texting me to refill them. Did you know that some of prescriptions include payments to doctors who prescribe them (Mitchell et al., 2021; Zarei et al., 2022; Sayed, 2024)?[1] After some more research, I got ideas about what to do outside of the medical industry to support my recovery and healing from this deadly disease.

Adding Dance Dharma *as Medicine*

Somewhere around June, that's three months into treatment, still in phase one of the intravenous chemo protocol, I wised up: *I'm going to dance. I can't just lie here or sit here and waste away.* At that resolve, I began dancing again. I danced to accelerate healing and deny illness. That's when the remarkable upturn in my health started.

Small moves first. Little by little. A minute or two at a time. Sitting up in bed and moving my arms like I was doing ballet, and holding my fingers as I had choreographed for a dance. Just a few motions. Smiling and dancing with my eyes. Choreographing the pain out of my body and into the dance. Then I'd add head movements to go with the moves—slowly at first; fast moves gave way to dizziness and I'd have to return to being prone. Making an infinity sign, then tilting my head as if I was in arabesque. Next, in that position, I did point-and-flex moves with my feet, ankle rotations, and *passés*, first on the right and then on the left. After that, some one quarter-circle *rondes de jambes* in the air, sitting and then lying on my back.

By July, with doing dance this way, I became strong enough to get out of bed for longer than a few minutes. I used a banister in our house as a ballet *barre*. Holding onto it, I started with a few *pliés*, *elevés*, and *relevés*, and low leg lifts, front, side and back. Soon, I took a chance on releasing the makeshift *barre*, doing some sacred dance moves, such as sweeping the arms, lunging forward keeping my spine straight, and making half turns, then lifting into *promenades*, in the center of the room while music played. Then sweeping arms in large circles with a rhythm, some head rolls, and expressive moves *à la* modern dance as I'd done in the past. Nothing high-impact and always careful not to twist or bend my spine. I tired very easily. I was so weak. These were true weights that I pushed up and through as I did dance. And for those moments the meditative aspect kicked in. I left the cares and concerns, and received assurance and love, self-compassion.

Around the end of September, with the infusion chemotherapy completed, some stamina returned and the mental fog lifted. I was actually dancing again, for maybe ten or fifteen minutes at a time. Many of the debilitating medication-related side effects and disease-related symptoms had diminished. I believe that, yes, the chemotherapy killed the cancer cells. I also know for certain that reducing that dose of oral chemo was critical. I also believe that had I not returned to dancing, my mental and spiritual health would have continued to decline, my weight to drop, and my body to weaken—even with the reduction of the cancer cells through chemotherapy. Chemotherapy, oral or intravenous, not only kills the cancer cells, it kills other needed cells, resulting in destroying the immune system and the will to persevere. All together, they hurt the body, mind, and spirit nearly as badly as the cancer itself. Please don't think I'm saying you should do this. I'm telling you my story and everyone is different. What I do know is that everyone has to be attentive to what they're doing for their illness, and not just submit themselves to the protocol.

Dance Dharma provides a way for us to find strength in those all-important aspects of body and mind. It builds on itself, builds confidence in our choices. It assures us we're loved and cared for in this day-to-day existence, knowing that what we can see with our eyes isn't all that is happening, not all that is there. We can feel ourselves getting stronger. And it doesn't matter what the dance looks like or what type it is. It gives us moments to focus on something beautiful and allows us to turn off our thinking, worrying, and fears. In other words, we drop away body and mind.

Needing More Care in the Care Team

The monoclonal antibodies injections (mABs) began at the beginning of September, and the intravenous chemo ended about a month earlier. These injections were to be weekly for four months, then twice monthly for a few months, then monthly thereafter. The monthly injections were to continue until the disease progressed, or got worse. Since this was going to be a long-term thing, I understood from reading that the care we receive, that is, the patient experience when diagnosed and treated with any disease, is important; people need to feel like their care team members personally care about them (Gawande, 2014; Avlijas et al., 2023). I wasn't feeling this way.

Around November, halfway through the weekly mABs, I opted to continue treatment at a different cancer treatment center, one that was closer to my house, and I wanted a lot more "care" in my care team. Through reading and researching physicians at the center, I was able to assemble a group of women physicians, from India and Africa, to work with me. Here they spoke to me as their equal, touched my body when examining me, didn't rely only on test results. The oncology nurses touched with tenderness and kindness. The nurse practitioners were calm and gentle, never in a hurry, never brusque. And where the previous care team stopped requiring a look at my labs before the mABs after the third injection, or premeds before the injection, the second team required both and would not administer the injection before the lab results were provided. It was important to do that, I came to know, as on one occasion at the end of the every-two-weeks protocol of mABs, dexamethazone, Benadryl, Tylenol, and the oral chemo med, my liver enzymes were extremely high, so the team refrained from giving the mABs and ordered an ultrasound of the liver and gall bladder. Thankfully, those showed nothing acute. With some research I learned that the liver is substantially negatively impacted by oral chemo meds, and these can cause liver disease as if it were cirrhosis or hepatitis. My new oncologist, Dr. D, said the meds could do this to some people. She turned away from me when she said it nearly in a whisper. At that point I stopped taking oral chemo all together.

At the second treatment center, there were warm blankets, and lunch offered if you were there over the noon hour. Like the other cancer center, the patients also mainly lay prone, caregivers sat still, and the only movement within the infusion room was the same. Each cubicle had a television for patients to watch, each with its unique remote control.

Zazen as Medicine

What I see now, after deeply diving into Zen Buddhism, and engaging with the practice realization it offers, is that often, ego keeps racism alive, stable, and afflictive in my mind. Stress weakens the immune system and MM is a cancer of that system, and when thinking about or experiencing racism, recognized or not, that stress is a cause arising from conditions. Which in turn, I believe, makes people more prone to MM and other cancers. As I've already said, everything arises from conditions and causes. Yes, I had a firm resolve to ignore antiblack racism. I'll admit that even the strongest resolve to ignore it, without a way to understand causes and conditions, doesn't prevent emotional and psychological harm from it. Causes are "when this, then that," or "when not this, then not that." A tremendous amount of "you're an American Black, so this then that" happens, spoken and unspoken. Without a viable skillful path to deal openly and directly with the strain, one can take an unskillful path, adhering to a mental state of victimhood. That path which is often the default mental position feeds the ego harmfully. There we generate more greed, hate and anger, and delusion.

Even facing this reality, the conversation about Buddhism geared toward people like me has absconded. On the one hand, Buddhist centers are generally predominately European or Asian led, and these leaders can't address antiblack racism directly with American Blacks, and on the other, we're not likely to embrace Buddhism, given that it's highly likely we don't know of it. In my case, I hadn't encountered Buddhism until 2018 when I visited Tassajara Zen Center for a guest stay. Besides, if some do encounter Buddhism, they're scared of engaging with it. Why? Historical beliefs and Christian teachings usually disallow trying other religious practices. Assuming though that we overcome that barrier, some may perceive antiblack racism at Buddhist centers. Thankfully, I didn't.

Zen Buddhism can address sores of racism that American Blacks and other people of color try to cover up and deny or ignore. It can also reduce stress, and in combination with movement and medicine, can support a better quality of life with or without cancer. Taking up the practice, we learn the role of the mind, we are not separate from others, intentions are the roots of causes and conditions, everyone is suffering, and our egos drive us to act, feel, and make judgments. It is important to offer Zen Buddhist practice as medicine to us, so that we know who we are actually, and at the same time, have privileged classes continue to be self-reflective and accountable to ending antiblack racism. By 2021, I vowed to follow that spiritual path by taking the Precepts, and engaging in what's known as *Jukai* with my teacher. At that point I became a Lay Practitioner. And I'm glad I did. Zazen helped me, along with Dance Dharma, to recover from my cancer.

Zen Buddhists focus on Zazen, quieting and stilling the mind, and cultivating kindness and compassion for self, and primarily others. There is no gain in Zazen. There is an aware, attentive, awakened mind. This practice along with the *Wisdom Paramitas* allows the conditioned ego to loosen its hold. For example, you might think, "God, they treated me like a dog. Or this doctor [insert person perceived to be in control of you] is totally racist." These kinds of thoughts, like the ones I had with the doctor asking me to take the drug test, can cause us to be stressed unduly, and contribute to cancer and other illnesses. Over time, that thought, and thoughts like it, can be dismissed, diminished, and devalued through seeing how the ego creates delusion and applying Zen Buddhist practices. The body and mind are both there, free from the constrictions and confines of acting from self: that you exist separately within in a culture, or that you're separate from other people, places, and things.

Attentiveness is about being in the present, to see things as they truly are,

> but to see this, to realize it, you have to do a lot of emptying out, unraveling the conditioning that you have and that you are actually burdened by. Your conditioning—your social culture and your traditions—none of this helps ... it's not clarifying the mind [Kwong, 2022].

Zen Buddhist practices help us get through what is and what isn't and see and decide what response we will have when self-imposed or historically imposed conditioned suffering arises.

Lying there in my bed nearly dead, as I said, I was full of sadness and grief, and there's nothing like facing death that brings it all right in your face. I did Zazen while lying down in my bed. I started asking myself questions when I felt shame and fear, like somehow this diagnosis was my fault. I read lots of Zen Buddhist books, and listened to podcasts, letting them teach me and fill me with Buddha Dharma.

After a while, I asked myself: What if I saw my life and its and cultural causes and conditions differently, as a contributor of continuing illnesses, pain, and sadness? To do that, I just watched the thoughts go by, and told myself don't act on them, don't believe them, don't cling to them. This is a way out of being attached to the racist system itself, of beginning a process of moving away from clinging to any racial position.

Understanding causes and conditions impacts on our lives can be seen when breaking everything down into their component parts, by inquiring into them (Nagarjuna & Dharmamitra, 2009). The idea is to refrain from attaching a judgment of any kind, just see thinking, actions, and behaviors without contributing a judgment. If you don't have any ego involvement, there is peace.

Putting the practice of Zen Buddhism in the front of my mind while I was lying there truly helped me devalue some of the mental trauma associated with a terminal disease. Of course, like I mentioned already, I also had a therapist but she wasn't working on my spiritual needs. Together, dance, meditation, and appropriate medicines resulted in a miracle of recovery for me.[2]

Before and After
a Cancer Diagnosis

Then things look like they're permanent and solid. I can't tell what's really going on.—Anderson, 2012 p. 115

Balance History

Dance Dharma and Zazen provided the support I needed throughout cancer diagnosis and treatment, and importantly, they provide a life raft to hold onto when everything you think you know is turned upside down. Establishing a daily practice of Zazen as I mentioned earlier can be a very grounding force when coming face to face with terminal cancer's question of life and death reality. That's why I believe it's crucial to get your practices going, or to fortify them if you already practice. Now, not tomorrow. Life is impermanent. As it is said, time is short, don't waste your life. It's important to know that what we're seeing and believing is necessarily accurate.

Now I'll admit history is what it is. American Blacks and other disadvantaged folks have a hard time in some instances getting good or any medical care. As we hold that truth and the influence of ego in the forefront of our minds, I'm going to give a brief overview of poor treatment of American Blacks when it comes to medicine. The point of doing this is to hopefully help you to be informed and assertive with your health, while you attend to the Zen Buddhist path before you. It isn't live one or the other, either embrace Zen or be forced into responding from the cultural conditioning of antiblack racism; you live instead from within the ocean of Dharma, and the *Wisdom Paramitas*. Live by vows, not by happenstance. My approach is to see events, now, then, and soon to be, and people associated with them, with loving kindness, equanimity, altruistic joy, and compassion. To accept that I have been conditioned and my mind, body, and life reflects it to a degree. It is also true that I reflect the path of Zen Buddhism too. Often it is necessary to put compassion first. Importantly, realize these four ways of seeing contribute to understanding self and others. With this having been said, I'll go over a bit of macrolevel medical history in the United States. I also delve into what American Black women, men, and children suffer as a result of antiblack racism, along with LGBTQIAP+ (lesbian, gay, bisexual, transgender, queer, questioning, intersex, asexual, pansexual) people. Once that's done, I get into ways to get medical coverage, and setting up your access to care. In the end, I suggest that being prepared and relying on Zen Buddhist and Dance Dharma practices help alleviate suffering, while encouraging us to remain in reality. I believe these all make for a better quality of life, and a way to keep our egos from pushing us into unskillful actions.

A Brief History of Medicine for American Blacks: No, It's Not Equitable

History tells us that American Blacks and other people of color have often received less than the best or timely medical treatments if any. That is still going on these days, too.

It is true that American Blacks, when they have received medical care, more often than not received substandard health treatments for centuries. As far back as history recounts, American Blacks have suffered from being considered less than human or human enough to be "guinea pigs" for trying out medicines. Black people were also employed by white medical schools to "resurrect" Black bodies for use in the study and practice of medicine. In being brought to the colonies by slave ship, many Black people died from lack of care, ill treatment, or starvation. During slave transports, Black women suffered more as they underwent horrific medical treatments and experimentation with no way to protect themselves. That began in 1619 and continued well into the mid–nineteenth century (Nuriddin et al., 2020). And for those who reached land in reasonable health, often their owners ignored any illness or defects, and instead demanded that people just keep working. This kind of conditioning still remains with us. People go to work sick, as they can be feeling they "have to." I wish this history was different for other ethnic groups, too, such as those of Chinese origin. The main thing that stands out for other people of color, at least in my mind, is that they were and are able to have their own medical professionals and didn't have to depend on whites. This is due to the fact that American Blacks were brought to the West, deposited on the shores, and had their being, personhood, sense of self, eliminated. Over time, the idea that they needed to assimilate continued to drive the way of being of dependency on a structurally racist system without any way to resurrect or replicate the one they knew before enslavement in order to thrive.

And yes, slaves were emancipated on June 19, 1865; it took years before the fact was known to many American Blacks. What we now have as a national holiday wasn't recognized until two centuries later. On June 15, 2021, the Juneteenth National Independence Day Act was signed, mainly due to the outcry after George Floyd's murder (see Wikipedia, *Juneteenth*).

During Jim Crow, structural racist policies informing health care systems kept American Blacks from being able to access good quality care, and the same was true during the Civil Rights Era, when the money was funneled to doctors and facilities to cover the gap between the cost of health care and the way in which the government funded those costs. While some American Black people were able to get public assistance to cover medical costs, doctors and facilities often charged more than what the government covered and in turn demanded that difference from the patient. This practice is still ongoing today, and isn't limited to government-sponsored coverage. More, American Blacks weren't employed in roles that provided health care insurance, generally, and they weren't in jobs that were unionized. So the bulk of the burden of the costs for treatment rested with the individual. Without a job with full benefits for health care, or a union for protection of the health care plans, many people were unable to receive equitable, let alone good, treatment, information, or resources to help them remain or get well.

> Structural racism operates through laws and policies that allocate resources in ways that disempower and devalue members of racial and ethnic minority groups, resulting in inequitable access to high-quality care [Yearby et al. 2022].

What are health care systems that rely on policies and laws now? Hospitals, emergency rooms, urgent care, nursing homes, addiction recovery centers, all doctors' offices, skilled nursing facilities or rehabilitation centers, physical and mental therapy, cancer centers, infirmaries, surgical centers, and so on.

Many examples of policies that erect barriers to access for good medical care for people of color include employer-sponsored health and dental insurance for those working a particular amount of hours, and marital status. You may be denied coverage if your spouse can't put you on their plan, if you have preexisting illnesses, or if you work less than the required hours in a pay period. The Affordable Care Act (ACA, established by President Obama) was enacted to help people who aren't married when their partnership wasn't recognized as equal to marriage, have no health insurance, work and earn less than a certain annual salary, and who may be working in a role where their employer doesn't offer health insurance. Even with the ACA being a stabilizer, still some health care policies and systems refuse to accept that insurance or the ACA itself doesn't pay at the rate the facilities charge for services, leaving patients to pick up the tab. When this happens, many will forego seeing a doctor or other provider. They don't have the resources to cover the gap or they remember perceived historical inequitable treatment.

And please realize, health care systems relentlessly pursue people who have not paid their medical bills, and, even worse, it's difficult for a patient to know what the costs will be before engaging in the treatments. It's a purchase for services where you don't know what the cost is before you buy, and unfortunately, in many cases, you've already signed a document that says you'll pay any difference. There's also no way to verify you got the treatment you paid for, good, bad, or indifferent, nor any way to "return" the service or get a credit for poor service. And if you don't pay, you can wind up with credit problems, and even have to file for bankruptcy protection.

Who Gets Good, Bad, and Really Bad Medical Care

Unfortunately, good medical care in the United States is generally only available for those with adequate health insurance or those with enough money to pay for the costs. Adequate health insurance includes choices for coverage for illnesses, as well as annual wellness evaluations, for everyone in one's family. These are mainly for people insured by their employer or who have the means to self-insure. If a wealthy person needs care, whatever it may be, they are able to travel to facilities inside and outside the United States to receive it. Or, they have the ability to bring the care to them, without any regard for the costs. Those without these options are poor people, or those earning less than a required baseline, regardless of race, and the numbers are frightful. Let's look for a moment at Black Americans and people of color, who are women, men, children, and those who are included in these groups *and* who self-identify as LGBTQIAP+.

1. Black women are dying more than any other racial group or ethnic group.

Historically, being forced into sterilization has been an issue. While some poor white women were in this population, American Black and other women of color were involuntarily sterilized. As a group, American Black women are at a severe disadvantage for health care access. Why? Two points to consider here. Not only are we lower wage earners than men, and yes, lower than black men too. We are the lowest of the low in terms of the structural antiblack racism that exists in this country for its citizens. Uterine fibroids, endometriosis, hysterectomies, lack of wellness exams and prenatal care, lack of cancer screenings, domestic violence, hypertension, and diabetes plague American Black women.

Part Two

Black women's suffering has been with us since the onset of slavery, and the ways in which it's kept alive through medical systems is heartbreaking.

> Across race and ethnicity, including Asian and Pacific Islander mothers, Latina mothers, Black mothers, and white mothers, [Black] women reported experiencing discrimination during childbirth. ... The findings showed better treatment among white women, English speakers, and those with private health insurance. About one in ten [Black] women reported being spoken to disrespectfully by hospital personnel. The same women also reported "rough handling" by hospital personnel and being ignored after expressing fears and/or concerns [Taylor, 2021, pp. 62–63].

In addition to these findings, Black women's average earnings are less and we experience higher unemployment and poverty than our counterparts. We are the head of household more often, with more people to support, living in racially segregated communities. There the property values are lower as well. Here we find discrimination in mortgage lending too. That discrimination is called "redlining," a legal practice that allows lenders to deny loans based on race. The long-term practice resulted in community disinvestment. Residential segregation causes racial disparities in health, operating through many social institutions (including labor markets and education), and impacts overall health and well-being (Chinn et al., 2021).

2. American Black women of course aren't the only ones suffering since slavery. In today's world, American Black men suffer from hypertension, stress, and the impossibility of what it means to be a Black male in the United States, in historical and current cultural representations. These in turn cause damage to their families, friends, and the communities they live in. Though not true, American Black men are described in many negative lights. While this isn't the case for many, even so, with these stigmas and stereotypes, American Black males are targeted for incarceration, brutality, and killing, through policy and practice. Within these contexts, American Black male medical care is sorely inadequate and unequal. "Black males' health disparities are not just a public concern; they are a national crisis trickling

---

down to Black communities around the United States" (Williams et al., 2020).

Nine out of ten American Black men live *without* being incarcerated or spending time in prison. All told, American Black men suffer from more illnesses both physically and mentally, arising from cultural situations generally, and difficulty constructing a sense of their own viable masculinity specifically, and have less access to trustworthy quality care or medical and dental insurance. Black men have the highest death rate, lowest life longevity, and highest duration of disease suffering in the United States.

This isn't the only narrative available to Black men; there are many American Black and people of color who thrive. "They thrive as they know the history focus differently, attending to acceptance of their ... heritage and a spiritual practice such as Zen Buddhism" (Lateef et al., 2024). And by extension, I believe this is also true for American Black women. That means we, collectively, as American Blacks, can change our point of view and affect our communities, families, and selves. A lot of this can be done in the practice of Zen Buddhist meditation where we examine our thinking and change its relation to egocentric structures. This can help children and families.

3. American Black children are also treated poorly in the medical system, and some of that comes from adultification. That's the way American Black children are treated as adults even before they mature out of childhood. They're expected to act like an adult, which comes directly from the history of enslaving, when often children lacked parental protections. American Black children are also dying more than white children, in part due to having high suicide rates. Researchers think that's a cause of, and outcome from, antiblack racism and lack of access to mental and physical health care, as well as to adultification (Gordon, 2020).

And as women were treated horribly from the beginning of slavery, should their babies be born and the women remain unsterilized, those babies were cast off to die based on eugenics: Black mothers weren't any good and the children were inferior or defective. As late as 1972, forced sterilizations were happening all over the United States, on American Black and women of color. The goal was targeting low-income women to reduce public assistance costs.

Just like I talked about earlier for Black women, where children live is also a determinate of their health, or what some call opportunity gaps. One study reported:

> We examined racial/ethnic opportunity gaps, defined as the difference in the score of the typical White child's neighborhood and the score of the typical minority child's neighborhood. For the 100 largest metropolitan areas combined, the Child Opportunity Score for White children is 73 compared with 72 for Asian and Pacific Islander children, 33 for Hispanic children, and 24 for Black children. ... Non–Hispanic White (39 percent) and Asian and Pacific Islander (40 percent) children are concentrated in very high-opportunity neighborhoods, whereas Hispanic (33 percent) and Black (46 percent) children are disproportionately concentrated in very low-opportunity neighborhoods (Acevedo-Garcia et al., 2020). There is also the fact that mental health diagnoses go unaddressed in certain populations, contributing to children's long-term poor health [Bitsko et al., 2022].

So, Black children suffer from a myriad of systemic and policy impacts coming out of a history of antiblack racial discrimination. Having the parents take up new ways of seeing without denying the facts is a very important factor for changing our relationship to behaviors and thoughts.

4. Before leaving this topic of who gets poor medical attention, I don't want to forget our LGBTQIAP+ (as defined as lesbian, gay, bisexual, transgender, queer, questioning, intersex, asexual, pansexual) human beings. They suffer "discrimination experiences ... among health care staff in health care settings. Discriminative behaviors experienced [by these] individuals were stigma, denial or refusal of health care, and verbal or physical abuse. Knowledge and educational levels, beliefs, and religion of health care providers affected their attitudes toward [these] patients and their homophobia level" (Balik et al, 2020). LGBTQIAP+ people are discriminated against, are violently attacked, and receive less than equitable medical treatment. For example, medications are withheld based on discriminative

beliefs of health care workers, and withholding is increased if the person identifies as American Black male, or is transgender. The outcome of all discrimination was to convince these populations to defer treatments, routine exams, and follow-ups while increasing addictive use of substances and other self-medicating ways. Those who have the option of keeping their sexual preferences to themselves do so, avoiding being discriminated against (Ayhan et al., 2020). The people in this population face tremendous negative treatments in the medical systems:

Trans people experience greater discrimination and high rates of interpersonal violence, while at the same time, fewer people in this population have medical insurance. Specifically, trans men ... people with the capacity for pregnancy are often excluded from breast cancer screenings or gynecological/obstetric care, often because medical staff make the wrong assumptions about the person's biology. Furthermore, the labor exclusion and poverty experienced by many trans women can lead them into prostitution, exposing them to a greater risk of incarceration, violence, STIs, and drug abuse. Among this sub-group, black and Latin American trans women are the most affected by this type of exclusion and are most susceptible to experiencing physical assault, sexual assault, and murder. In addition, lesbian and bisexual women have a higher risk of not having access to cancer screening services [Medina-Martínez et al., 2021, pp. 2–3].

Black People Weren't Complicit

These examples of historical medical antiblack racial injustices, along with others, prompted responses from Black communities "who challenged and actively subverted racist structures in medicine to care for their health. Time after time, White dominance was rejected and alternatives were proposed. While health care remained segregated, Black communities established, funded, and operated hospitals in underserved areas. Black physicians established the National Medical Association (NMA) in 1895 to address the fact that the American Medical Association didn't allow them to join. Black hospitals and medical schools like Howard University and Meharry Medical College provided medical education and training when Black physicians were barred from other institutions.

Black physicians, nurses, and students led the charge for the desegregation of medical institutions for the benefit of staff and patients. Tuskegee Institute's founder Booker T Washington originated the National Negro Health Week in 1915 to focus on the poor health status of Black populations" (Nuriddin et al., 2020, p. 951).

Writing history with a different lens, in *Certain People, America's Black Elite*, Stephen Birmingham (2024) gives a social accounting of wealthy American Blacks who attended a private preparatory school led by Charlotte Hawkins Brown and were offered entrance into university education upon successful graduation from her school. During the early part of the 1900s, they were given a different narrative on how to be in the world. And there were many of them, coming from across the United States. While the school offered Negro History, the curriculum excluded Negro spirituals, with the founder believing their messages reinforced slavery. The curriculum emphasized being completely assimilated into white structures of society. Dr. Brown intensified some of the class ills found in American Black society, such as elitism, exclusion, and separating the haves from the have-nots. My point in bringing this forward is to open us to the fact that there are different realities, different reactions, and different rejections of the trajectory of slavery among American Blacks. Although many had issue with the road and path described by Dr. Brown, many of those wealthy American Blacks who lived in the United States played and still play a significant role in displaying how self and the understanding of self, the resulting narratives we tell ourselves and others, can lead to different outcomes.

Now in this current century, we still see so much disparity, again what was displayed during COVID, and the quality of treatment delivered to American Blacks and other people of color. We also see the denial of treatment and health coverage to LGTBQIAP+ people, and the villanization of people, or the de-biologicalizing of human beings. There is also a concerted growing policy and social effort to deny American Blacks entry into white U.S. medical schools (Sausser, 2024).

Rest assured, if people of whatever ethnicity have the financial means, they can get whatever they want done to their bodies. In any case, it's up to American Blacks and other people of color, regardless of their status in terms of gender or social class, the individual as well as the collective consciousnesses, to act and think for themselves. In turn, this affects others, as we aren't separate as we are conditioned to believe.

How Can We Influence the Antiblack and Racist Systems?

Changing thoughts and behaviors is what practicing Zazen and Dance Dharma can do. That means of course we have to let go of some ways of being and adapt others. Zenju Earthlyn Manuel, an American Black woman and Soto Zen Buddhist Priest, gave a Dharma talk recently at Green Dragon Temple (Manuel, 2022). In it she brought in the notion of how to understand causes and conditions in this way: *How are you the chaos in the world,* she asked. What she meant by this chaos, I interpreted to mean how are *you* the continuation of the problems arising from causes and conditions that are disempowering? Like antiblack racism, bigotry, poverty, war, climate crises, and so on.

Her question resonated with me: I want to take up a very politically incorrect question, how are we are creators of and sustaining of some conditions of antiblack racism? Before going on, let me say that the ways antiblack racism came about had to do with greed, hate, and delusion. Africans sold other Africans to traders, who shipped them to colonies. It's a terrible history, subjecting so many to egregious atrocities for a long time. Those left and still leave psychological karmic scars on all who live in the United States, not just American Blacks. Let me also say that there is no simple "Black American community"; we are diverse within different social, cultural, and economic strata.

In her Dharma talk, Manuel referenced *The Mis-Education of the Negro* (Woodson, 1933/1999), in which the author averred that if someone's thinking is controlled, their behavior is easy to control. If you make a person believe they are inferior (or superior) you don't have to make them do anything, they will seek behaviors aligning with their thoughts. American Blacks, like everyone, often continue suffering by keeping their minds replaying conditioned mental tracks and holding dear the belief of self in the forefront. Changing the mental tracks requires the ability to let go of the cultural constructs in the psyche to relieve suffering, to loosen clinging to identification of what one has been told.

The mind and the underlying ego are at the center of it all.

Some American Blacks, from all socioeconomic strata, support belief in Christianity. That's not an issue, and Buddhist practices can be complementary to it. What may cause difficulty, though, is some also revel in remembering how badly we've been or are being treated, and at the same time themselves fall into bigotry. Across the culture it's expected that American Blacks cling to a show of solidarity. Many believe they are owed support and exceptions from other American Blacks as well as society, claiming they are victims. It's so easy, nearly considered natural, to place blame and take a position of a different kind of entitlement. At the same time, there is social pressure to stay within the cultural system, to enjoy all media's portrayal of Black culture that parades suffering, keeps stereotypes in place, and speaks the language derived from being in it. That means accepting unskillful ways of being that are harmful. Leaving this system is seen by many as an act of treason really, and those who do are degraded with an intracultural kind of hate, greed, and delusion. And that kind of thinking is precisely what cultivating a practice of Zazen and Dance Dharma can change, allowing reduction of suffering and different ways of interacting in the world.

In summary, we have a history of problems in medical treatment. American Black women, men, and children are deeply impacted and so are people in the LGBTQIAP+ groups. In addition to taking up the practice of Zen Buddhism and acting in the ways described by Zenju Earthlyn Manuel as I detailed above, we have to know and remember that there are people who aren't complicit and act in ways that stand to change cultural conditioning.

From a changed viewpoint, one way we can possibly advocate for more positive outcomes is through attending to stressors that have cancer and issues related to it held at bay before they emerge. In addition to the *Eightfold Path* as ways to bring about a more favorable reality, in the next section I talk about advocacy for yourself, all the while assuming that Zazen and Dance Dharma have been taken up as practices so that debilitating beliefs can be set aside so that the best available care can be had. For the remaining pages in this chapter, I offer some practicalities that may be of benefit for you and your loved ones navigating the health care system.

At a Medical Service Visit

The first thing you encounter, after establishing your insurance and identity, are forms to fill out for medical services. Often you don't get to read them. They're coming to you electronically or being shoved in your face when you're waiting to see a health care provider. People want you to sign them on faith. Instead, ask for the forms to be printed out, or if you're doing it at home, read them carefully. Many people don't know they should print out the agreements and read them, and they are reluctant to do that, or ask at the time of treatment. By then, they are typically in an acute situation. I've heard that uninsured people aren't likely to do wellness visits, like getting an annual physical, precisely based on not having insurance. So using the emergency room or doing urgent care becomes the safety net of a nonexistent health management process. It's skillful to follow a wellness visit plan, and in each case, read the documents carefully. In addition to agreeing to pay for any balances not covered by insurance, the documents also say they'll share your health information to folks.

What I've learned and what I do is print out the forms, draw a line through the wording that I don't agree with, and initial and date it. As written in an article for doctors and health care providers called *Medical Informed Consent*, "[P]atients should be made aware that they are allowed to strike out any part of the medical consent form with which they do not agree or to which they do not consent" (Paterick et al., 2008, p. 316). Yes, this takes time so that I'm not passive. This is what I consider to be Right Action on the Noble Eightfold Path. Then, when I've completed the forms, I sign them, and I ask the people at the desk for a photocopy right at the time. If there is a surgery involved, I do the same thing, including what I want to be done for emergency blood transfusion, organ donations, and the rest. If I can, I try to do these at preoperational appointments if they're offered. When they aren't, you're sitting there getting ready for surgery and they're putting all these forms in your face. You have to read them. You have to take time and do it before they give you anesthesia.

If your doctor comes up with something they want you to do, like a test or something, such as a stress test, some kind of biopsy, or a scan or what have you, it's critical that you validate the actual need for it. If you have insurance, beware of doctors just using up your insurance to bill for more even while you may not actually need the test or whatnot. If you don't have insurance, ask about grants and financial support provided by the institution. Many resources exist. The difficult part is doing all this *before* any procedure. Importantly, getting wellness checkups and annual physicals can reduce the need for an emergency room (ER) visit and gives you agency over your care.

At the same time, if your doctor ignores your symptoms, it's important that you get a different doctor. In any case, review all the forms and don't be afraid to cross out anything you don't agree with.

All of this fits with the need to be attentive to causes and conditions, that is, if this, then that. Being present with your health, taking good care of yourself, is self-compassion, and compassion for others. Doing it in a way that allows for you to be balanced, or have equanimity, is being loving and kind to yourself and others. At the moment, we can remember the history of medical treatment of American Blacks and resolve to put aside the ego's prompting about how it was, stop the focus on the inequities that means therefore we should be fearful and angry, which contributes to being further deluded. As you sit Zazen you realize that you let go in order to allow turning your life in skillful directions, not only in medical care. The turning includes living within many systems and policies. I suggest coming from this perspective to address cancer treatment, or other life-threatening treatment, when interacting with the health care system.

Access to Cancer Treatment Isn't What It Seems

To fully live, getting these aspects of care arranged and established before a diagnosis allows us to be ahead of the curve. Cancer can be both very debilitating and deceiving. In many cases, if found, it's diagnosed late in its progression, which means our capacities are diminished. This can be true for many types of cancers. When cancers are diagnosed, there can also be errors in the diagnosis, and the methods for treatment may vary. This is why getting a second opinion is important. Of course, the sooner you get an accurate diagnosis, the sooner treatments can begin. No doubt, with each visit to see a medical professional there are medical costs. And there may be a lack of qualified American Black or people of color medical professionals where you are. So getting your team set up and identified, or your plan arranged, is extremely critical.

Start by getting basic health insurance for yourself and children if you're in a low or no income category.[1] Then search for a primary care doctor. Go see several doctors before you decide on one. You may have to visit a few before you find one that you feel comfortable with. When you have settled on one, go for annual checkups and scheduled wellness visits. Get all the routine health and wellness screenings. These are usually at no cost. Ask to have your blood looked at for cancer indicators in addition to the routine blood work.

Identify the cancer treatment centers near you. The treatment centers can be what are called community, regional, or national. Go online to search for them, and review the oncology doctors they have. Familiarize yourself with them before you have a diagnosis. Check to see what kind of insurances they will take. See if they have grants or other support available for people without full coverage. This process can be tedious, so doing it before you're debilitated is a skillful action.

If you do have a diagnosis of cancer, and your care team, which your primary doctor likely will refer you to, or the cancer center you found, sets up a plan that includes medicines and other treatments like chemotherapy, please read the information. Ask questions. Ask what the treatment plan is. What are the costs? Find out if there is financial assistance available. What are the risk factors? How long will the plan take and how does it cure the cancer? Ask for all the resources, from social workers, therapists, support groups, and dieticians, to people who will come and clean your house, take you to your appointments, and so on. They are available for cancer patients. These may not be voluntarily offered to you. Ask, ask, ask.

For your cancer, find out what the issues are, and what the impacts will be if you take or don't take the medicines. What is the life expectancy? Prognosis? You may find that doctors are reluctant to tell you and instead they'll evade the question and tell you about averages and median longevity. Just know they are averages, and remember that there is a wide universe that is supporting your life. It wants you to live to help others as well as yourself.

In my case I was given the three-stage protocol of infusion, bone marrow transplant, and monoclonal antibodies for the incurable MM. I read the information, researched online, and determined to forego the bone marrow transplant not only due to my risk factors, but also based on quality of life concerns. Remember that you're the one in the driver's seat when it comes to your health. My commitment to my practice of Zazen and Dance Dharma helped me to keep my resolve. The doctors will give you information and you'll need to ferret it out and make decisions. Lots of times the protocol is just a method parsed for everybody, not necessarily for you particularly. Don't ignore the history of American Blacks and the treatment received in medical systems, and at the same time don't let it hinder your proactivity and compassion. Don't let your ego tell you negatively what's not there. Some of it is. Consider though that in lots of cases it's just delusion. Look clearly at reality. Let the *Wisdom Paramitas* be your guide. Your life isn't only for you, it is for others too. That's why it's all the more important that taking care of ourselves is a critical aspect of living a life that isn't based on self, not driven by ego, grounded in Zazen and Dance Dharma. If you aren't attentive and present, taking the *Four Noble Truths* and the *Noble Eightfold Path* into your daily interactions, some clouds may cover your eyes and prevent your clarity.

---

5. Before and After a Cancer Diagnosis

At first, the diagnosis will overwhelm you, and then the medications may make you feel like you don't want to do anything. You may feel like your life is without meaning or you wasted it, or so will many other thoughts arise that are pretty normal if you face such a point. You'll have to rely on your practice to remember who you are. Now, I'll go over some ways that you may support yourself with a cancer diagnosis to enable a better quality of life even while you're dealing with a deadly disease.

A Better Quality of Life

Please know that *Dance Dharma* and Zazen—based on your physical abilities—improves our lives, may also reduce the need for medicines, and contributes to the quality of life for those with cancer. You can take part in Dance Dharma and Zazen no matter where you are, in a bed, in a chair, or on your feet. I've already given instruction on Zazen in these three aspects: lying on your side, sitting in a chair or on a cushion, or doing *Kinhin* as you walk slowly. If you're unable to walk, you can certainly do Zazen sitting or lying down. How about Dance Dharma?

Yes, you may dance in a chair or in bed! Whatever dance you like. Get some music going if you can, maybe use your cell phone if you have one, and some headsets. If you don't have that ask for someone to bring you something to play your favorite music on. Make sure you're not disturbing people if you can. Turn on the music, and move your body, whatever part of your body you can, whether your eyebrows or your pinky toes. Move them, smile, and take in the present moment. Of course you can move without music too if you prefer. Please don't forget you can also watch dance and receive a valuable benefit! Find dances on YouTube or on your social media pages that you relate to. You can also copy some of the moves as you sit or lie down, and if you're able you can do them yourself.

In addition to doing Zazen, surround yourself with inspirational readings or recordings. If you have your cell phone, look for some podcasts with Zen Buddhist Dharma talks or download audiobooks and ebooks on Zen Buddhist practices. Choices abound to help you stay or continue your practice, and to ensure yourself compassion, and compassion for others. You can check out YouTube for some very inspirational talks and discussions on many aspects of Zen Buddhism. Online groups that sit Zazen are accessible to support you, too.

One thing I found that was helpful was setting a time each day to do these helpful movements and meditations. Just like you have to take medicines at a particular time each day, think of these movements and meditations as medicines. I did and still do them more than once a day. It only takes a few minutes, whatever you can do. If it's possible, maybe ask some folks to join you. Dancing and meditating together creates a sense of connection for you and the others around you. It fills your space with healing and hope. Even if there're not dancing and meditating with you, you keep doing it anyway.

Now Is Different

A cancer diagnosis is a life-changing event. It makes you see things about yourself and the people around you in different lights, maybe helps you to make a new resolve about what's important to you and what isn't. Family and relationship dynamics come into play. If you were the one taking care of everyone else, they'll need to figure out how to do that for themselves. Or on the other hand, if you have unresolved situations with people, you'll want to get them rectified. Here's a place where resentments and estrangements will come up and need to be addressed. Children, significant others, parents, employers—all will have come into your consciousness.

I relied on the Zen Buddhist way of living to help me with the people in my life. I think it was realizing that I didn't want to leave the earth without attempting to smooth out any unresolved causes and conditions. I started with my mother, then moved to my son, then my husband. I tried to share with them that I loved them and cared for them, and wished them well. I came from the place of loving kindness, altruistic joy, equanimity, and compassion. I understood that they suffer and I let them know that. The thing was, I didn't expect anything from them and it was a skillful way to be. They didn't change! They still kept being who they were and I let them be. Of course at the beginning when you tell your loved ones you have terminal cancer, there is a bit of an "Oh no!" that comes out. They'll ask what your prognosis is, how much time you have to live, stuff like that. Some people won't be able to handle the news at all and will want to run away or avoid you, or say things like "I'm so sorry, anyway, as I was saying...." Some will say "Let me know what I can do," knowing there's nothing they can do. Being around and near people who are safe, and who are interested in you and your well-being, is the key. We all know that many people talk too much and don't listen. Now more than ever probably, that's what you need, people who are safe to be around, who don't talk too much and who are interested in listening to you, or being silent with you.

Setting boundaries with loving kindness is required with all people in your life, even before you have cancer, definitely after a diagnosis. If you don't want something that's being offered or you feel forced to accept behaviors, remember you can limit any negativity. One reason for this limiting is the importance of reducing chronic stress—stress that arises from "reasons like adversity, depression, anxiety, or loneliness/social isolation can endanger human health." Chronic stress is stress that is ongoing and hurts the body and mind. That stress is a very big deal in cancer, and there is some evidence of it being linked to some types of cancer.[2] Many American Blacks and other people of color face heightened chronic stress during their lifetimes. Therefore, it is critical to address the fact that chronic stress can make life more difficult, can put you in mental states that are unhealthy, which no one needs, particularly not after a cancer diagnosis. Chronic stress management therefore becomes very critical in taking care of your health.

A variety of ways to alter chronic stress are out there, like focusing on breathing, slowing down, and of course meditating. I found that practicing Zazen and Dance Dharma are important to get the body and mind moving, while also incorporating chronic stress reduction practices. Know there are other ways too. One is to remain present and attentive as you connect movement to your daily activities. If you reach for a glass of water, remember that you're dancing, not just moving. As you eat, remember that you're moving, dancing the move, not just taking it for granted. Slow down and focus on breathing and breath. When you find your mind drifting to fear of the future or thinking of negative thoughts of the past, focus on a mantra. One mantra that I use is "I take refuge in Buddha, Dharma, and Sangha." Many mantras can be found that you can memorize to shift your thinking. Small prayers are wonderful for this or longer ones if you have the memory for them! Prayer beads worn on your wrist are also helpful. As you finger each bead, say a mantra or a prayer.

Gratitude also helps. Make a gratitude list every day. Try and be creative so that the list extends from being grateful for food, clothing, and shelter. Think of small supports that you have. A bed, a chair, people who care, clean water, a warm bed. Whatever you have, a beating heart, fingers, toes. The ability to move and meditate. If you can, hold the focus of being compassionate to yourself and others as a perfect gratitude. Be grateful for calmness that comes from managing stress. Celebrate any good news, no matter how small, and of course at all times be grateful that you're kind, that you can be kind to all those you encounter even when you feel agitated.

Hurry is a killer. We've been hurrying too much to get away, get ahead, and get by. Slow down, take time for what you need. Be more clearly present, get enough sleep and rest when you need to, don't give in to languishing and laziness. Fatigue will dog your steps; overcome it daily by moving unhurriedly. Focus on the now, knowing that today is when you have, where your body and mind are realizing the active process of enlightenment.

The final areas of this chapter that I'd like to cover have to do with moderation in healthy eating, watching the news or being on social media, and physical isolation. Even if you were following a healthy diet before your diagnosis, it's really important to keep that going or start if you haven't been. Find moderation in foods that are prepared well, at home if it's possible. Avoid eating out, eating processed and packaged foods, or eating fast food. They're generally loaded with extra salt and fat or sugar, and/or have extremely large portions. In many cases they cause chronic inflammation, which is a stress trigger for the body. These can cause heart disease, cancer, diabetes, obesity, and digestive interferences. Focus on getting enough low-cholesterol proteins, like chicken and wild-caught fish, or tofu and high-protein plant-based foods if you're vegetarian/vegan, and enough fiber, such as whole or sprouted grains, beans, and fruits and vegetables. Drink plenty of water. Though I love bacon, I had to let it go, and reduce eating beef and white bread, and foods that cause chronic inflammation, which is associated with cancer and other debilitating illnesses.[3]

I found that reading or watching too much news or being on social media was stressful. Everyone on social media has something to say and often, intentionally or not, it makes for greed, hate or anger, and delusion. Each day there are stories about adverse events happening to American Blacks for no reason, LGBTQIAP+ folks getting mistreated, and so many other reports that just keep the chaos going, as Emanuel suggested. That doesn't mean to ignore the world's conditions; it just means find a balance. Pick a time of day, maybe once a day or once a week, whatever works for you, to watch the news or scroll social media.

In this chapter I've given you an overview of my preparation for dealing with cancer through my practice and realization of Zen Buddhism. Next I talked about some history of American Blacks and others who have received poor or inadequate treatment within the health care system. It was also important to know that not all American Blacks were from impoverished backgrounds, and the way the mind works has a lot to do with one's reality. Again, this is not to say that antiblack racism doesn't exist nor to imply it's not a problem. Then I discussed what to expect at a medical visit service visit, and to understand the ramifications of cancer treatment. Zazen and Dance Dharma, and self-care with people, foods, and media, are important to improving the quality of your life during cancer treatment as well as outside of a diagnosis. Finding a middle way as you walk this path is a prescription for your cycle of life and death and ultimately, planning your transition from that cycle of embodied life. This latter point is what I discuss in the next chapter.

6

Planning for Transition from Embodied Life

Speak well and softly give at all times
Benefit each myriad thing and person and situation
Have no space or sight for discrimination, for greed, hate
and delusion through the cycle of life and death
                            —Tanahashi, 2013, p. 476

Death Isn't a Topic of Conversation

In my childhood home, death was all around. It wasn't talked about. People were killed by violence, out in the street or right inside their homes. Family fights, domestic violence, settling a dispute, being initiated into a gang, were all means of killing. Using guns, knives, or hot grits. People generally didn't call for emergency personnel or report homicides. There was no use; protective police and emergency medical resources weren't allocated to that for American Blacks in my childhood neighborhood. When people heard of someone dying due to illness, it was chalked up to their not having good medical care. I already covered some of problems with access to care in the previous chapter. Suffice it to say that there's a real history of this, and I've already suggested ways to address it.

Still, death as a topic was broached at church funerals. Or maybe in a sermon or a bible study when talking about the idea of going to hell or heaven or an afterlife when one dies. Or the example of Jesus's resurrection put forth the claim that death is a temporary place, and that if one is obedient, resurrection was for them too. That theory was very abstract and in a sense put the topic "out there" somewhere with nothing to really help with understanding death, why people and other beings, such as our pets and animals, appear on earth and then disappear. In my world, families didn't talk about death, and many had deep, strange, emotional responses to deaths: maybe sad, maybe glad. Maybe supernatural. And at the time, grief therapy was out of the question, if it was even something to consider, from the cultural stance against the need for mental health counseling or the availability of it.

In other practices and within some of the Black Christian churches too, people saw death as something that gave freedom to human spirit beings, or provided us with phantoms and ghosts that haunted or guided us. In my childhood home, my mother was convinced that people died and their spirits entered other living people and newborn babies—a kind of reincarnation, so to speak. Before they settled down in another body, they came back to the family and tried to get attention. Lots of people thought this way. For a child, any of these beliefs and theories could provoke fear of death. That fear persists up and down the social scale, in many communities, regardless of ethnicity and income.

You'll hear people also say they're not afraid of death, and some will wish for their death as soon as possible. They want to escape the pain of living on earth that includes disparate treatment, poverty, drug addiction, or just being alive and uncomfortable in their skin—fearful of how life is where they live, seeing the unfairness of it all. Let's not forget the terminally ill or the aged who would just like it to be over, as they're tired of their bodies and minds and the effort needed to stay alive.

Then there are those who are so afraid of death they don't want to hear about it or consider it.

As we age or encounter sickness, the work required to care for the body becomes more obvious and often difficult. Going to get lunch isn't the same, getting a shower isn't the same, or driving isn't the same. Over time we may become unable to take care of our daily chores and activities, plus we may need assistance with every little task. Not only that, some of the most feared aspects of aging and illness have to do with loss of mind, decision making, and autonomy.

And without our really talking about deterioration, dying, or death much in our culture in the West, these changes, when they arrive, take us aback. When they hit, we need to have the means for health care where in many lives there is little to none. Instead, over our younger days much of our attention was directed to beauty, sex appeal, eating, drinking, fashion, overexercising, getting pleasure, gaining fame and fortune. Distraction from the impermanence of the body, believing in being separate from the world we know, and having an ego driving point of view is what I call it. It's what the media and culture do, and why turning off the television and social media are so important (Hahn 2002). And in our families there is an increasing trend of moving away from seeing or helping elderly members decay and die. Instead they're placed in assisted living or nursing homes, a whole hugely profitable industry unto itself, to be looked after by others. Dying and dead bodies aren't our thing. There isn't a comprehension of where the liver is, or the lungs, or the pancreas, as examples. We don't talk about the body as being in a skin that envelops organs, veins, bones, and brain. Bodies are decaying until they reach the grave, and they continue to decay until they decompose and return to the elements.

Speaking of graves, in certain areas, they're mostly "over there" where we set them, out of sight and out of mind. Yes, some visit the grave sites of loved ones, or we attend graveside burials when someone dies. And of course there's cremation and maybe a celebration of life ceremony. Overall, gravesites are out of sight and out of mind, ignored as we ignore what to do with our bodies in the process of when they completely stop working and stop breathing. We leave it here on earth for someone to handle it.

In his book *Being Mortal*, Atul Gawande (2014) gives us a good look at how our bodies deteriorate and what to expect as they do, as well as how to deal with the medical profession as we age and die of diseases. He particularly treats the topic of terminal cancer with detail that helped me see my way through the medical system, to ask the appropriate questions, and to make extending quality of life decisions. Medical personnel aren't really able to talk about death either. Mainly their job is to keep people alive, even if it's not a quality life.

In Zen Buddhism, we are encouraged to see our bodies as deteriorating objects and to take care of realizing the cycle of birth and death.

On Birth and Death in Zen Buddhism

A newborn baby comes into the world, met with joy or disappointment, depending on the circumstances. Into whatever circumstances they are born, babies aren't always seen as the opposite of dead people or in the context of a life and death cycle. In lore, you'll hear someone say one person dies and another person is born. In our American culture birth and death are considered and set in dualistic terms: One is good, the other is bad. No doubt, in Zen Buddhism, birth and death aren't separate events, one isn't valued higher than the other. They are nondualistic, equally valuable, and beneficial. And we don't think of a soul that goes from one body to another after the body expires. Why? Simply, the Buddha didn't teach that, even though some Buddhist traditions will discuss karmic reasons for rebirth and give guidelines about what to do to prepare for death and returning to life. Instead, in Zen Buddhism, there are no promises of a heaven or purposeful placement into hell. A considerable effort is made to realize we don't know what actually happens at physical death, nor anything about how consciousness is placed in newborns. In the end, each practitioner must work out their understanding of life and death, and must understand that without the two, one can't actualize the Buddha Way. Taking refuge in Buddha, Dharma, and Sangha is a skillful method to keep the focus on what your life and the lives of others mean. We say that each person embodies a radiant light that is worthy of respect. That includes those we have issues with, and ourselves! Each day is important to remember life and death. This is an opportunity to know you're here, as you have been somehow fortunate enough to have a human life. We're not to waste it, waste it on chasing after anything that just causes more suffering, realizing that everything is impermanent. Death is always there even though we usually ignore its presence or are so distracted by looking outward at the world. Death's presence helps us realize what is critical, helps us to be wise right now.

It's very necessary to arrive at death having worked deeply on your life, to know what it means to be human, and how that humanity is practicing all the precepts, taking refuge in the Triple Treasure, and living by vow. To be able to help others through the *Four Noble Truths* and the *Noble Eightfold Path*. In a short phrase, practice the way of a Bodhisattva.

Birth and death are happening each moment and are continuous. Each complete breath is one cycle of birth and death. So paying attention to our breath is to study the meaning of birth and death. Sitting Zazen is practice for realizing birth and death. We sit as still as we can, not moving for an itchy ear or a slight feeling of touch on the top of the head. Unless it's absolutely necessary to move (like if we have to go to the restroom, or we feel sick, or there's an emergency in the Zen center), we sit in Zazen letting go of our bodies and minds. Not thinking, not solving any problems. Being human, emotions come up though while we're sitting. We remember something from the past or have some kinds of fears arise. When that happens, I look at the root of that thought, and I can always trace it back to an ego position, connected to me not getting what I hoped to gain, or losing something I had gained, or feeling like I'm right somehow in a given situation. And further, when I consider how I got to the place that put me into that situation, I can trace it back to going too fast, being in some kind of desperate circumstance, or being greedy or angry. And importantly, assuming everything is permanent. Take, for example, when you go to a concert or other event and you have a good time. Maybe there's a lot of laughter and you feel good. As these emotions are happening, perhaps the thought arises that you'd like to do this again. Suddenly, there's a shock wave, like for instance COVID, and it's not possible to recreate such a feeling. We're grasping onto it, looking for ways to make it happen again. Of course, it's not possible. Then we feel bad, and try to hold onto the memory even tighter. We feel like we didn't do something right, or we should have done something differently. The main reason for the concert attendance was to escape from the day-to-day drone of living, looking for excitement, maybe thinking about sex, having something good to eat. That's all about escaping suffering, driven by ego's belief that this will make you feel better. Now, it's okay to go to the concert as long as you understand that it too is impermanent and will not change fundamentally your position within life and death.

Being free from birth and death, living as a Bodhisattva and a Buddha is the purpose of Zazen. It's being emancipated.

> The Great Way of all buddhas, thoroughly practiced, is emancipation and realization. "Emancipation" means that in birth [life] you are emancipated from birth [life], and in death you are emancipated from death. Thus, there is detachment from birth-and-death and penetration of birth-and-death. Such is the complete practice of the great way. There is letting go of birth-and-death and vitalizing birth-and-death. Such is the thorough practice of the great way [Tanahashi, 2013, p. 450].

Emancipation for American Blacks is freedom from enslavement—all types—and erasure of antiblack exclusionary practices and other types of discrimination. To experience emancipation within life and in death in the Zen Buddhist context is to live fully in each moment, at one with our activity with appropriate responses. The purpose of Zen Buddhist practice is finding emancipation and realization by understanding our minds and egos. That is, we realize that birth and death are just continuations of our good fortune to be born, to help others, and with the opportunity to truly understand the nondual nature of continuation through birth and death. Zazen allows us freedom from grasping and freedom from aversion so that we don't grasp onto fear of life or death (Weitsman, 2008).

The Buddha's teaching emphasizes reducing desire, or transforming our lives from Samsara, suffering, to Nirvana. We like to think that birth and death are opposites, and that if we avoid death we can reduce our Samsara. Though for some people life and death mean transmigration from life to life, for practitioners of Zazen they mean absolute freedom to enjoy Samadhi, a peaceful life of nonduality. Life and death are the Buddha. There isn't anything to fear, nowhere to try to get to, to avoid anything. That realization is nirvana right now, rather than nirvana "over there somewhere." It's the great relaxation from the total anxiety humans feel when they come to know that birth and death are one. That means every human being knows that death calls. As a Zen Buddhist, the Buddha Dharma is that we aren't dealing with the duality. We are dealing with the oneness of the continuation of practice in life and in death. To realize that, the important thing is to stop searching for permanence. Life and death are the full expression of Buddhahood. Knowing this, we make the best use of life and death. What this means is that we realize everything in the present moment, stop engaging in delusion.

When lying on a death bed, it might be too late to begin the work to evaluate the importance of birth and death. I was there on my death bed, in so much pain that physical movement was nearly impossible, and with little capacity to exert any mental force. The medications made me drift in and out of consciousness. There was no conversation with my inmost self available. Just before that stage, I had the ability and the motivation, for about an hour each morning, to go through my personal matters, to clear out nostalgia papers and documents, damning photographs, letters, and, to send what I thought would be helpful to my loved ones. As I drifted between consciousness and unconsciousness my thoughts kept turning to the relationships I had with people, especially family members. I'm not sure how your family is, but in some there are estrangements, feuds, blaming, disappointment. Having a terminal health condition doesn't necessarily mean everyone will suddenly change their points of view, their habits, criticisms, or be able to be less self-obsessed. For me, I thought it was necessary to connect with my immediate family and let them know what was going on. It was a difficult decision; I'd rather have had them not know. I felt that way, supported by believing there was an off chance that I would recover and there'd be no need to let them know. I also didn't want any of them to visit me as I was deteriorating, and bring dysfunctional energy into my space. After all, I was dying and I wanted to make sure I left no trace of negativity as the transition of body and mind occurred, from life to death.

It was also on that supposed death bed that the awareness of antiblack racism came pouring into my mind. At the same time my experiences and witnessing American Blacks' poor treatment of each other through learned bigotry nauseated me more than the chemo meds did. I allowed the sadness, powerlessness, and the unfairness of it all to come into the forefront of my thoughts. The jobs I didn't get selected for, those who wouldn't publish my writing, the ignored or disrespectful treatment I received when I did get hired or published, inflated interest rates, how the judicial system didn't actually provide justice in many situations. And how the educational system fails us. All of these and more haunted me.

Just about a year prior to the diagnosis of MM, I landed a prestigious role, which would turn out to be the antiblack racism icing on the cake experience. It was a great opportunity, I'd thought, to get some recognition and prestige. That wasn't what happened. Instead, I was ostracized. What happened? What had I done? I discovered later that it wasn't me.

There was an antiblack racist person who didn't like American Blacks and who also held sway over the community. Someone informed me that the person warned anyone who'd listen not to acknowledge me in any way. That was someone who was a generational member of several pre-Civil War Southern social societies, and was also a large donor in the community. They would pull their support from anyone who acknowledged or worked with me. It was just like when other people of color were threatened by people in power if they served, sold to, or catered to American Blacks. Turn them away or you'll be put out of business, or worse, you'll be unable to live comfortably.

After a bit of introspection, I conceded yes, the way they acted was hurtful. Also, and most importantly, I finally realized what I'd done, over and over in my life. I was clinging to an idea driven by my ego. In reality, I was just a speck in the wide universe, desiring fame like many of us, mistaking it for love and acceptance. Over the years I did what many American Blacks do—persevere. Doing so, I worked and relied on people who wanted to work with me. And there were many, and I'm grateful for them, of various ethnicities.

Having all of these feelings surface as I was lying in bed, sick and tired, angry, ashamed, and feeling like a failure, a thought occurred to me: What if I looked at all situations as arising from my ego? What if I looked at them as Dharma Gates? What if I looked at them as causes for my suffering as if they arose from a deep desire for fame and gain? What if I was coming from the place of greed, hate and anger, and delusion all the time?

The same question came up when I thought about what I'd seen in American Black bigotry toward others, and the ways some people in an American Black community steal, hurt, kill, put others down, and are self-centered, never thinking of others and never considering living by vow. In it a mirror of a racist society emerges, a copying of what has been done to them, sacrificing awareness, living from a deluded point of view. Having been cast aside and belittled for centuries, left out and ignored, unable to have nice things, being poor, being tricked into debts that could never be repaid, having been used in medical treatments against their wills, and so on, it's really no wonder that there are bigoted American Blacks. It's what we've been taught, what we've experienced. And with their having not been exposed to Zen Buddhism, it can't be sorted out any other way than to have compassion for them.

Now, as I've said before, racism and bigotry are painful no matter what. It would be nice if people could give them up. In the end, they don't make suffering less, they don't help others, and in fact they're causing more harm. And in no case do I mean to imply that poor treatment on any level should be accepted as okay. What I'm saying is that often the circumstances are prompting us to act unskillfully as we claim that they are "unfair."

Whether we agree with the unaware action taken or not, seething with anger inside will not help our life and death stream. It won't allow us to see that we are fortunate to have this life, as it is the way to emancipation from life and death through practicing and realizing Zen Buddhism. Every single irritation and feeling of anger is from the ego, from wanting something, gain, fame, recognition, fair treatment. Loosen the grip on those wants, let them go. Keep letting them go. And then, find some ways you can do something, little somethings, to help assuage the greed, hate or anger, and delusion. Do it to help others, forget about getting anything. Even though we are socialized by Western values to "get something," it's a trap. There isn't anything to get. We are on the life death train, and getting off of it depends on realizing the trap, by letting go. And let me say too, there's nothing wrong with having a nice life built on the *Noble Eightfold Path*, and following the Precepts. Choices made with these in mind also will put that ego in the right place and bring it to the right use. This allows us to take ourselves off the center of the universe and place our gaze on the Way. It's imperative that we not waste our lives being distracted by unimportant ventures. How we address and meet the transition from life to death, how we are emancipated within them, is critical.

Setting Up a Will

Once we have been emancipated from life and death physically, our bodies remain on the ground of earth. Its elements will lie as the empty object that it is, decaying and smelling, with no sight, sound, smell, taste, feeling, or consciousness. Nothing to do, nothing to attain. No fame and no gain. There will be nothing known except an object decomposing in the universe on the surface of the earth. Someone will need to look after it. If we have any material goods or other objects, someone will need to look after them as well—unless you want the governments to take over handling your estate. The emancipation and transition leave the body unable to do a single thing on its own except decay. No one will be able to hear your answers about what you want done with your belongings, or your assets and liabilities, how you want your body disposed of or why you were the way you were in your life. Someone may be able to infer what you may have wanted. It's a good idea to leave this information in writing. While only a very small percentage of American Blacks and others of color have a will and trust (death is hard to think or talk about), setting one up and having it notarized is the skillful way to care about others who have to manage your decaying elements, your assets, and your liabilities. "Few people understand the hoops and hurdles their loved ones will have to navigate at the time of their death if an estate plan has not been executed. Kenneth Kelly, Chairman and CEO of First Independence Bank stresses, 'We need to make what I would say are wiser decisions in terms of taking care of our loved ones'" (Christian, 2022).

Even if you feel like you don't have any assets or liabilities, still this is an important aspect of life and death, a final communication that you leave for people who will care for your elements after you have gone on. It also ensures that you keep your financial assets within your social and family groups, rather than allowing them to fall to the city, state, and federal governments where they will be used without acknowledgment of the gift you made, inadvertently. If you don't have a will and trust, each state has its own laws governing your assets and liabilities. All liabilities will be paid first, and whatever's left will go to your heirs, in a particular order: usually the current spouse, children, then others.[1]

It's true that a will and trust can be contested by people, and that family arguments can tie up a will for decades, making it impossible to execute. This fact does not obliviate the need to make it. If you can, hire a trust lawyer and work with them. They are easily found by doing an Internet search or talking to your friends who can make recommendations. Recently we learned that some American Black people neglected to set up wills, such as Aretha Franklin, leaving all her family to sort it out among themselves, and, with that, the intervention of the state and federal government. Prince, Bob Marley, Barry White, had the same situation. American Blacks aren't the only ones. Howard Hughes, Pablo Picasso, and others were also in that boat. We can't ask them why they did that. All I can imagine is they must have had a reason, or, they didn't want to face the fact that one day their bodies would lie on the earth without a pulse or breath.

If you don't feel you have the resources to hire someone, you can go to the library or search online for a sample last will and testament.[2] Make a list of the things you have, and fill in the items on the document to fit your situation. Assign a name to whom you'd like to bequeath each object, whether it be a friend, family member, or foe, or an organization. Next, type up your list and take it to a notary public. Then once signed you'll want to place it somewhere that people can easily find it.

Of course, if there are no assets and no friends or family, the state will provide a simple burial. If no one claims your body, the burial will be held in a public gravesite and paid for with public funds. If you have debts outstanding and no assets to cover them when you die, your family members may be responsible for them and pursued by debt collectors for paying them back just as if they were theirs.[3] For these reasons, and probably others I've not spoken about, the loving and kind skillful action is to take care of these details before you're unable to get them set down on paper.

Arranging What You Want—Resuscitate Orders? Hospice? Assisted Living?

As you prepare your last will and testament, you'll also assign an executor for your estate, prepare for a power of attorney, a resuscitate directive, organ donation directive, and so on. The phrase "executor of your estate" doesn't mean you have a lot. Or, it could mean that. Here the term "estate" simply includes the items you consider important, and they can be anything. The "executor" is the person you trust enough to make sure your wishes are upheld after your body becomes its unmoving elemental object. Questions like what do you want done with your organs, that is, do you want them donated to science, will need to be answered and written down. Do you want to be on life support if you're suddenly taken to the hospital and rendered unconscious? In other words, do you want to be on breathing machines or other intubation equipment to keep you alive? You'll need to state this clearly. The default without a directive on this matter is for medical authorities to keep you alive whether you're conscious or not. Your person who you selected as the power of attorney can make the decision to take you off life support for you if you haven't clearly stated your wishes in the document, or if you can't be brought out of a coma.

If you're conscious as you walk through the end-of-life transition, where do you want to be when your body transitions? At home? In a medical facility? In an assisted living establishment? Leaving these decision to later or to someone else is a bit risky. First of all there are costs associated with each one of these choices. Do you have long-term disability insurance? Or long-term health coverage? People under 65 years old need to have these in place. At 65, Medicare can cover some costs, but maybe not nearly all of them. Having taken out insurance policies at a younger age can help defray costs, though as we age the policies can become too expensive to retain.

Engaging hospice can happen at your place of residence, in a hospital, or in assisted living facilities. In my case, I'm choosing to stay in my home, and bring in hospice care when it's needed. Everyone has to make their own choices. I have witnessed family members and friends in assisted living facilities, and I learned that people have to have considerable savings, insurance, and resources to ensure their coverage. My choice isn't based on that alone; it's based on the fact that being in your home is the amazing, loving, and considerate way to leave the body gracefully (Gawande, 2014; Hensley, 2021). Some people disagree with this based on their position in the medical system. In any event, dying at home allows a place of familiarity, gives greater ease as there is little disruption, and it's easier to control who comes and goes into your space. Dying at home is wherever your home is, regardless of the location. Hospice care comes to you, as do other technicians and providers. And yes, it is true that there is distrust of the medical system by American Blacks; still, hospice at home can alleviate the generally more intense suffering experienced in a hospital (Farmer, 2022).

After having spent some time on these details of planning for you transition, it's equally necessary to bring to light which people you want to include in your space to support your transition.

Creating a Team of Folks to Support Your Transition

In 2022, there were about 224,000 American deaths from cancer and nearly 74,000 of them were American Blacks. According to the American Cancer Society (2019) we have the highest mortality and the lowest survival rates. And indeed, the rate of MM diagnoses is on the rise.

Matthew Gavidia (2023) found that over two thousand deaths from MM happen each year, and American Blacks make up 20 percent of all new cases and 18 percent of total deaths per year from MM in the United States. Stated differently, one in every five patients diagnosed with MM in the United States is an American Black. Moreover, according to the American Cancer Society (n.d.), African Americans have more cancers and have greater barriers to cancer prevention, detection, treatment, and survival, due to policy issues and lack of health insurance, and of course antiblack racism. Black people have the highest death rate and shortest survival of any racial/ethnic group for most cancers in the United States.

Even though at the moment no one knows what causes MM, nor how long you'll be able to live should you be diagnosed with it and receive timely and adequate treatment, being intentional about who you'd like to support your transition is critical. That's also a true mental point of view for any cancer or disease. Leaving it up to chance may mean you have individuals around you that you don't like or don't appreciate. This ranges from caregivers to friends, family, professionals, and loved ones.

Asking someone to be your caregiver is huge, especially since death and dying aren't really in the forefront of our culture. Also, it's a responsibility that is seen as overly taxing and stressful. As well, being a caregiver is expensive (Worthington, 2024). Asking or allowing someone to be your caregiver means they'll do a lot of chores for you, covering your day-to-day life management even if you have hospice care or in-home health support from professional aides and therapists. Being a caregiver can be isolating and stressful, especially for American Blacks. Many caregivers feel like they have been forced into the role. And sometimes those who receive the care from people who were "forced" feel like they're not being treated well. In one example from my family, my aunt had lung cancer. Her son was living with her all of his life. He'd long been ignoring her wishes for what she wanted in her home. When she got terminal lung cancer, he was the one that was there all the time. She yelled at him from her bedroom, trying to get him to comply with her wishes. Little things like take out the trash, or go to the store and get so and so, were ignored. Instead, he played cards and dominoes in the living room with his friends. You get the point, and yes, I know not all situations are like this. If you can, avoid having a reluctant and recalcitrant caregiver by identifying those who are willing and able, and you can create an atmosphere of greater calm. A different relative, for example, my uncle, had this situation when he was diagnosed with stomach cancer. Though he died soon after his diagnosis, his wife was his caregiver, with lots of in home health support. When it came time, all of his wishes were honored, including the details in his will. Whoever becomes your caregiver or caregivers, make sure they are fully aware and participating in caregiver support groups and training programs ahead of the need. If you can ask for and receive agreement from several people to help you, rather than relying "automatically" on people like your children, family, and friends, that would be beneficial.

As to your professionals, I already talked a bit about hospice. These supporters and providers need to be identified as soon as you can, even if you're not ready for hospice. So many choices for care clamor for your business, and many organizations out there promise they'll come to your service. Listen, though, it's really critical to call and talk to them, meet with them, get a feel for their culture and service levels. Hospice providers have become a nationwide network of delivery, asking for you to select a city and state where you live to determine who will be available. Your medical team works with hospice when you decide you're ready. They'll coordinate medications and palliative care. And when you exhale your last breath, they'll be the ones ensuring calls to the appropriate authorities and working with the coroner. Importantly, they'll also work with your loved ones and family to help ease grief. Your identified power of attorney, which I spoke of earlier, will also need to know who you have chosen for your hospice care and your spiritual leader, as your will and trust will need to include not only the details of what you'd like done with your assets and liabilities, but, as importantly, the disposition of your body for cremation or burial.

Part Two

In the case of feeling at the moment of having no one to identify for critical support, and no one that you can leave your belongings to, I'd suggest that creating a network before your need for people is critical. Joining in with structured activities and groups that do some of the things you enjoy would be a start. Make some connections so that you aren't just alone and by yourself. As Zen Buddhists say, everyone is interconnected and we rely on each other. Lots of these connections have come from churches in our culture. Nowadays that's not always the way to go. Reaching out and getting involved, volunteering at nonprofit organizations, especially those that have a mission to help others, is really nice. Join your city's chamber of commerce and get involved. Children who need to be read to, teachers that need a classroom aide, pets that need temporary homes, children that need guides during family courts are waiting for you. Let's not forget folks experiencing loss of homes, domestic violence, and of course hospitals need volunteers. Embracing and acting upon these numerous ways, plus others you may think of, to get involved and make friends, helps ensure that you're not isolated and alone.

Now if it's truly too late for that, and you have no one to turn to, your professionals and chaplains, your spiritual leaders, will be your support. They'll do their best to comfort you and befriend you.

Facing death isn't usually seen as a pleasant endeavor in our culture, at least before we learn and accept death as part of life, as a way of being in the world, and not knowing why it occurs or exactly what happens when we exhale our last breath. "Not knowing," as Zen Buddhists say, is most intimate. It's okay not to know the particulars of what happens as life becomes death, or to hold onto views that are unskillful. We're told that this life and death cycle we're on is one of opportunity—to practice realizing what this world truly is, without being captured by fear. Looking at it directly though gives you added freedom, allows loving communication between you and your circles of friends, family, and professionals, and mostly ensures that when the time comes, you'll be all set.

Being Clear About Your Surroundings as You Transition

Just as you identify what you want done with your belongings and assets, and arrange your team of folks to help you with transitioning from life and death, establishing who and what you want in your surroundings is also necessary. Of course, this aspect is needed particularly when there is a disease or old age that is the cause of death. With accidents and other tragedies, that is, at work or in a social setting, in a moving vehicle or a fire, or with stray or intentional bullets, for instance, that lead to your transition, of course you may not be able to direct where you wind up. Generally, humans transition due to natural causes. So getting your surroundings ready seems like a good move.

What do you want your space to be? The bedroom? Living room? Family room? Your studio apartment? What do you want it to include? Pictures? Mobile devices? Books? Music? Clothing? How about statues and daily readers? Prayer beads? Television? Think about being unable to move very far from your bed. What to do you want to be able to see each time you look around? Furniture? Wall art? Statues? Do you want particular blankets and pillows? Letters and cards from loved ones? Memorabilia? Flowers and plants? Pets? Razors, toiletries? Makeup? Grooming items like scissors, tweezers, clippers? And what do you want clothing wise? Shoes? Hats, beanies, scarves, wraps? Any jewelry? I ask about all these to support having what makes you feel loved near you. This helps you to feel grounded and at home in your body and mind. You'll need minimal stress and anxiety, and maximum stability.

Next, make a list of people you want to visit you during your last days. You can have anyone you want, or you can exclude anyone you want. You don't have to have a reason or justify your visitors list. Your hospice caregiver and power of attorney if you have one will be the enforcers for you. I know for me I don't want certain people around causing too much drama and angst for me. They live a lifestyle that isn't the same as mine, and while I love them, I need my space peaceful. And some people don't want any visitors, and still others want a Grand Central Station of visitors flowing in twenty-four-seven, and that's fine too. Just be clear about it.

Finally, do you have plans for a burial or a cremation? Please include the details of this information in this area of your wishes. What do you want your body to be covered with at burial or cremation? What do you want in your burial casket? Making these known by writing them down makes it easy for the hospice nurse to initiate and complete the arrangements for you and communicate with your family and loved ones.

Place the Documents on File

Now that you have your will and trust, your power of attorney, all your support team and your ideas for what you want your surroundings to look like, and who can be in them, you'll need to put the documents somewhere. Your power of attorney may be a good choice. Try to find others too that you trust to give a copy to. They don't have to have a copy of the will and trust. Consider that since you won't be available to answer any questions, they do need to have copies of everything else.

I've covered a lot of areas that people in our Western culture and many American Black cultures don't talk about in pleasant conversation or otherwise. Death is often feared and shunned rather than embraced and welcomed. Our understanding of why we live and die is often limited at best. Whatever we know, whatever we believe, one day our body will lie motionless and breathless. We can leave it unattended, and let others make their guess as to what should be done with it. The same can be said for any assets we have. As American Blacks we have the power to say what we want, even as our life flows into and beyond death.

7

Remaining Open, and Continuous Practice

[W]e indeed have no other life, no other place to find the Dharma than here ... in lay life.—Rutschman-Byler, 2009, p. 830 of ebook format

Over the course of these pages, I've shared much of myself and many personal experiences with you with the intention of helping you to see your life and the lives of others with a radiant heart and clear eyes through a lens that is different from what we've maybe known. That lens is Soto Zen Buddhist practice and Dance Dharma. Any benefit received as a result is dedicated to the Buddhas and Ancestors throughout space and time. My further intention has been to share these with you without any aspiration for gain or fame, offering you a way to clarify the ego and its conditions as related to and formed by antiblack racism and bigotry. In that context, seeing everything and everyone as connected to you at all times, giving you some means to view life and death, and ways to practice are really key within this book. There is an urgency here that I discovered during my initial encounter with multiple myeloma. And by the way, at this writing, I have no trace of cancer in my blood or anywhere in my body. Do I think this is unusual? No, I think it's quite normal.

The fact that we are here on this earth at this time and that you've read this book is auspicious. We are all imbued with this great choice: to pay constant attention to the aspiration for enlightenment, through life and death, and to help others realize it. We move with it, dance with it, meditate with it, evaluate causes and conditions with it, and finally live by vows rather than living by reacting. It's a different way of seeing, a different way for certain from the antiblack racist lens.

With a human life we have the greatest opportunity to practice and realize the Buddha and the Dharma with our bodies and minds. For me it is critical to notice this daily, rather than being automated and swept away by structural causes and conditions that create antiblack racism and bigotry. I watch the action like clouds passing through the sky. At the same time it is really essential to realize the impact that these antiblack messages have on my daily life, and to respond appropriately in any given situation. An appropriate response isn't always a mealy-mouthed one; every now and again it requires particular words that people can understand, or actions that don't always make people feel good. Even while acknowledging these points—living by vow, responding appropriately, etc.—I have to realize and remind myself continuously that I'm not separate from anyone. We all live in this ocean of life and death together, along with Buddha Dharma and Dance Dharma, and the people and products running the medical systems.

Recently I came across an article that shared stories about the shortage of doctors and the increases in employing nurse practitioners to fill in for them (Melby et al., 2024). What was shocking about the content of that article, I learned that many nurse practitioners train in online courses that lack the necessary rigor for meeting patients' needs. They aren't receiving the kind of knowledge that a person would receive in medical school, or even in a real-time, on-ground nurse practitioner program. As I stated already, in my experience, the nurse practitioners that treated me at the first infusion center weren't skilled in the area where I needed them—would expect them—to be. At the time, I didn't know that there was this kind of education being offered. When facing an illness or a routine medical exam, I've learned that just going along isn't always the best medicine. At the same time, some medical schools in the United States are blocking BIPOCs from entering (Sausser, 2024). As a practicing Soto Zen Buddhist, it behooved me to investigate and make changes that I could.

At the start of this book, I talked about culture and what it means in various aspects, and reflected on how these influence our beliefs and behaviors. Everything from addictions to cars to education and work have in impact on who we think we are, forming reactive stances coming from ego. Rather than continue on this train, living by vow, the *Wisdom Paramitas* and realizing the *Four Noble Truths* and the *Noble Eightfold Path* were introduced. They provide a perspective that frees us from reactive stances. These help us see the reality of suffering and move toward reducing it. They also allow us to open our hearts to see that others are also suffering, and, we are not separate from life, which is totally impermanent. Once we've done some exploring for ourselves internally, and come to understand ourselves this way, we can begin to present ourselves in a new light within our human interactions in our families, communities, and places of employment, helping others to see as well.

In detailing the Buddha's teaching on the *Four Noble Truths* and the *Noble Eightfold Path*, I went into discussions on emptiness and impermanence and steps to take in order to live by vow. By embracing these actions I proposed we find the power to live in a way that provides agency through our Buddha Natures, for all of us who have culturally conditioned behaviors that make for feelings of powerlessness. Next, I moved into Dance Dharma, or Dancing No Self, or Dance as Buddha Nature. These, I said, were part and parcel of First Nations movement practices. I presented information that shows how dance is very healing and supportive of health, and is itself a nonverbal meditation practice. I called it Theodance, and I then incorporated these ideas into the Zen Buddhist movements in some of the *forms*, or rituals we practice, and in mudras. After this connection of Theodance to practice realization, I went into detail about sitting Zazen, which is also a mudra of the full body, an active Dance Dharma done with a detailed choreography. When there is more than one period of Zazen, or at other times if appropriate, a dance called *Kinhin* is done. This is a form of slow walking. I discussed the Buddha's Awakening, and the Bodhisattva path. Then I talked about how to see birth and death differently than many in our Western culture conceptualize it.

In Chapter 4 I shared my personal story on how I relied on

Dance Dharma and Zen Buddhist practice to help me overcome MM and deal with the health care system. That system has been one that has historically had antiblack policies underpinning it, and that history still informs some of its practices. Dance Dharma and Zazen were both "medicines" for me. I believe deeply that these two medicines facilitated and aided the pharmaceuticals that were prescribed for the cancer and that I agreed to take. I also deeply believe that without my practice, I would not have been able to see the cycle of birth and death so clearly, nor the connection between causes and conditions as they appear in antiblack racism, nor seriously raise the need—take the risk to bring it—for American Blacks to have an exposure to Zen Buddhism. This is a whole medicine for helping healing and change for boundless numbers of people.

It's important to get to practice and realize it as soon as you can. Right now the alarm is sounding. Why? We live in impermanence. Know that when the body and mind are failing, as in receiving a fatal diagnosis, you won't likely have the energy to do it. Doing it before that gives you something to hold onto.

Then, in Chapter 5, I talked to you about BIPOCs and their health statistics over time, and presented some evidence of what kind of impact cancer is going to have in the future. It's not a pretty history or a rosy picture. American Black women, men, and children and LGBTQIAP+ beings often suffer egregiously from lack of quality health care, especially those living within poverty. Anyhow, the uncovering and dismantling of the ego from the Zen Buddhist perspective can help us today and tomorrow. This isn't the whole picture. Many American Blacks took action to create better lives and better access to education and health care. Let's continue to assert ourselves on the one hand, let go of being victims in causes and conditions, and also on the other hand, realize the history in order to do so. I give specific guidance about how to be assertive during a medical service, how to prepare for getting treatment before you're unable to, and how to establish a better quality of life after a debilitating diagnosis.

In the final chapter I got into detail about reducing antiblack racist anger, deeply contained in the ego, facing death, and making the practical arrangements for it. In our society death isn't something we like talking about, though in each moment of our lives it hovers over us. When we arrive at death, we won't be as afraid if we look at it differently with a dropping of body and mind, and see it as a continuous cycle. Being free from birth and death is the point of living by vow contained in the Buddha Way from a Zen Buddhist perspective.

This is the life I have. This is the life you have. We have to live it in a wholesome way. The fact that we have a body means we have the opportunity to realize our Buddha Nature, and to help others realize theirs. Dance Dharma, Buddha Dharma, Zazen are here for you. Do not let a mind of antiblack racism and bigotry hold you back.

8

Support for Your Dance Dharma, Zazen, and Medicine

[Buddhist] methodology assumes that the activities of the mind are the decisive factor in determining our well-being.—Hee-Jin Kim, 2000, p. 109

In these next pages, I share with you some ways that may benefit you in supporting your Dance Dharma, Zazen, and "medicines" for your life and those around you. They include, of course, Zazen, Dance Dharma, reading, reciting inspiration, and engaging with a practice group. You may also like to include some of your own practices as well. Having a schedule helps. All of this right effort begins with the mind and engages the body. I like to have daily, weekly, monthly, and quarterly aspects to my practices. I also find that there needs to be a balance between solitude and Sangha practice, either online or in person. That means finding the middle way that helps you and others.

Health care, mentally and physically, is critical and so are support groups to living a peaceful life. Some of those resources are included here as well. These help in so many ways, so please avail yourself of them. Suffering can be assuaged and we don't have to be alone in our recovery from cancer. We can engage our bodies and minds in skillful ways as we connect to our letting go of ego and self.

Daily Practice

Zazen

Getting your Zazen done before too much of the day has passed is a skillful way to begin. Maybe you can find a quiet place in your home or wherever you may be. Set up a place where you can be still, either sitting on a cushion or in a chair, or lying down. If you're in a hospital or nursing facility, it may be that someone comes in early to give you medicines. Set up your space so you can do this, before or after they attend to you. If you have work you do at home or otherwise, it's also a skillful practice to do Zazen before you leave the home or get online. Try to do Zazen daily if you can, and if you're just beginning to practice, take it easy. Maybe five minutes to start out with, and over time increase the time. Focus on your breathing and posture. Just let the thoughts come and go. If it feels okay with you, maybe you can do a few bows when you conclude. If you've been exposed to Zazen and have a practice already, you can add in taking refuge in the Triple Treasure, and of course saying other chants if you feel inspired. Often you can find online participation in services or recorded chants. Check out the San Francisco Zen Center's website; it has several posted.

Reciting

These suggestions are here for those who are beginning this practice. It would be nice if you could engage each day in the Loving Kindness Meditation (https://www.sfzc.org/files/daily_sutras_Loving_Kindness_Meditation). Why? It helps to shift our focus, helps us to begin dropping the held tight belief that we are separate from each other.

LOVING KINDNESS MEDITATION

This is what should be accomplished by the one who is wise, Who seeks the good, and has obtained peace.
Let one be strenuous, upright, and sincere,
Without pride, easily contented, and joyous.
Let one not be submerged by the things of the world.
Let one not take upon oneself the burden of riches.
Let one's senses be controlled.
Let one be wise but not puffed up and
Let one not desire great possessions even for one's family.
Let one do nothing that is mean or that the wise would reprove.

May all beings be happy.
May they be joyous and live in safety,
All living beings, whether weak or strong,
In high or middle or low realms of existence. Small or great, visible or invisible,
Near or far, born or to be born,
May all beings be happy.
Let no one deceive another nor despise any being in any state. Let none by anger or hatred wish harm to another.
Even as a mother at the risk of her life
Watches over and protects her only child,
So with a boundless mind should one cherish all living things. Suffusing love over the entire world,
Above, below, and all around, without limit,
So let one cultivate an infinite good will toward the whole world.
Standing or walking, sitting or lying down, During all one's waking hours,
Let one practice the way with gratitude.
Not holding to fixed views,
Endowed with insight,
Freed from sense appetites,
One who achieves the way
Will be freed from the duality of birth and death.

Mantras

Mantras are also positive ways to help focus the mind. If you're inclined, start by taking refuge in Buddha, Dharma, and Sangha, especially when you feel agitated, afraid, and wanting. One example:

I take refuge in buddha
Before all beings
Immersing body and mind
Deeply in the way
Awakening true mind
I take refuge in dharma
Before all beings
Entering deeply
The merciful ocean
Of buddha's way
I take refuge in sangha
Before all beings
Bringing harmony

Part Two

To everyone
Free from hindrance

As I mentioned already, if you're attending Zazen in person or online, some have recitations and chants included in their services. On many websites the words are available as downloadable or paper documents.

Dance

If you can dance a few times a week, that would be beneficial for the body and mind. For those who are able, use your whole body to dance and let go of yourself and everything else. Look for adult or senior dance classes in your area, or try to find them online if you live in places that don't offer them. A lot of community centers, colleges, or others offer them. And go if you can, even if you don't have a partner.

If you're not able to walk or stand, dance in your chair, or in bed, with whatever part of the body that you can, your eyes and head.

Start by moving the feet and hands. Do some rotations of the ankles and writs. Then if you can, do a few head rolls to the left and right. Don't go too fast on the head rolls so dizziness doesn't get you confused or nauseous. Next, lift your arms overhead, together a few times, then one by one. Try to get the arms to lie flat on the bed if you're lying down, or raise them to next to the ears. Hold them there before you bring them back by your sides. When you move, resist, think about moving them through water. Try to find a good pace, not too fast or slow. Then open your arms to the sides, and cross them back together, giving yourself a big hug. If you're able, then make some sweeping circles, as large as you can with your arms.

Next, try some leg lifts with side swings to the left and right. Lift your leg, whichever one, hold it out in front of you then gently move it to the outside then cross it back over the body to the other side. Alternate your legs one at a time, then see if you can do them together. Then you can do some toe and heel taps, in place, or extend your legs to the front and sides of your body.

When doing these dance moves, make them beautiful, add your own rhythms and timing. Try to realize your center and keep your back erect.

Don't forget your face! If you can, raise your eyebrows, both together and at the same time. Do some very large smiles, move your eyeballs left and right, up and down. Open your mouth and act surprised! Smile when you move your arms and legs.

You can make the moves flowy or snappy, or you can vary them. Remember to breathe and exhale deeply while you dance. If you'd like you can use music. Doing the dances in silence is also beneficial.

And of course you can read and practice from *Sacred Dance Meditations: 365 Globally Inspired Movement Practices* (Walter, 2020), which gives dance movement meditations for each day of the year.

Mental Health and Dance Therapy

Finding a therapist can be helpful with a diagnosis of cancer or other disease. They can also help to uncover ways to support a sense of well-being. Many therapists operate in person or online. You may have to try a few before finding the one who works for you. An Internet search will benefit, and you can also search on *Psychology Today*, or ask your physician for a referral. You can also check out some options provided by *Better Health*, https://www.betterhelp.com/advice/therapy/is-video-therapy-effective, which offers support in many ways and may offer free options. The website takes you through a questionnaire. It is best to be as honest as you can. It will ask you if you want a therapist that is BIPOC or what have you. It will, after you fill in your responses, ask you for your information to create a password and login. Then you'll be given options of therapists.

The *American Dance Therapy Association* has a website that lists qualified dance movement therapists, https://www.adta.org/find-a-dancemovement-therapist and so does *Psychology Today*, https://www.psychologytoday.com/us/therapists?category=dance-movement-therapy. Each lists them by state so you'll need to start there. Some appointments can be made virtually.

Studying Zen and Buddhism

Reading about Zen Buddhism is an uplifting support to practicing. Try to read each day a few pages or a chapter. Some references to books are provided below.

Excellent resources for studying Zen and Buddhism exist and are easily accessed. Here, in the first section are books, and the second section provides some online resources. Please know these are just a few offerings. If you do an online search for books on Zen Buddhism and other Buddhist practices, the results may be overwhelming.

The books listed here are a place to start.

a. Background Reading

Shunryu Suzuki, *Zen Mind Beginner's Mind; Not Always So; Branching Streams Flow in the Darkness.* These three books offer the thinking of the San Francisco Zen Center's Founder.

Thich Naht Hahn, *The Miracle of Mindfulness.*

Charlotte Joko Beck, *Everyday Zen.*

John Diado Loori, *The Still Point.*

John Daishin Bukspazen, *Zen Meditation in Plain English.*

Kazuaki Tanahashi, *Enlightenment Unfolds.*

b. Understanding the Bodhisattva Way

Robert Aitken, *Mind of Clover.*

Reb Anderson, *Being Upright.*

Daine Eshin Rizzetto, *Waking Up to What You Do.*

c. Theravada and Insight Buddhism

Bhikkhu Bodhi, *In the Buddha's Words: An Anthology of Discourses from the Pali Canon.*

Walpola Rahula, *What the Buddha Taught.*

Joseph Goldstein, *The Experience of Insight.*

Gil Fronsdal, *The Issue at Hand.*

---

d. Tibetan Buddhism

Pema Chodron, *The Wisdom of No Escape; When Things Fall Apart.*

Chogyam Trungpa, *Cutting Through Spiritual Materialism; The Myth of Freedom.*

e. Buddhist Information and International Resources

Buddhist Studies Virtual Library (http://www.ciolek.com/wwwvl-buddhism.html).

Sotozen Association (https://www.sotozen.com/eng).

Places to Practice Zazen
and Engage in Further Study

Practicing Zazen can be done in person and/or online. Many Zen Centers and monasteries offer both. Please do an online search and read the schedules of Zazen, and see if they work for you.

- San Francisco Zen Center (sfzc.org) includes Tassajara, City Center, and Green Gulch monasteries, which are Soto Zen lineage centers under Shunryu Suzuki. Branching Streams (https://branchingstreams.sfzc.org) is a good resource for finding affiliated Sanghas around the world and in the United States
- Zen Mountain Monastery (zmm.org) is located in New York, and is a Rinzai practice center.
- Plum Tree Village (plumvillage.org) is multisite, and international, and follows the practice of Thich Naht Hanh.
- The Buddhist Society of Western Australia (bswa.org) follows the Theravada Tradition.

There are many locations for study. Searching online will help you find places that will likely give you options. It's probably a wonderful opportunity to check them out and see how they resonate. Many of these centers also have podcasts, where they post Dharma talks. If you do a search on your device, you'll find them. All of those listed above have podcasts and many have apps to listen to. They are usually donation based.

_____

Teachers

Finding a Zen Buddhist teacher or other Buddhist teacher is an important part of developing your practice. It's important that you connect with a teacher who is "Dharma transmitted" in the lineage. That means they have been correctly ordained and are qualified for the role of helping you. The best approach is to attend the Zen center offerings before asking for a discussion with the teacher. Each Zen center will have teachers who are willing to meet with you in person or virtually to explore this important relationship. Take a look at their websites to find the listings.

Medical Access, Patient and Caregiver Support

Medical

The truth is that medical care for cancer is expensive and may be challenging if you don't have insurance. That said, most hospitals have financial support, such as grants, or other ways of "writing off" the costs. Always ask to see a financial counselor. And always try for the best treatment center you can find. *Cancer Care* also offers some financial assistance (https://www.cancercare.org/financial_assistance) so that you don't have to be without care.

Cancer, Caregiver Support, and Hospice

Cancer Care offers a variety of support groups (https://www.cancercare.org/support_groups), specialized by cancer type. Support groups are for both patients and their surviving loved ones and family, and caregivers. Nearly all the hospitals and cancer centers provide access to support groups, so please ask your care team for referrals. You will need to ask if the information isn't provided.

For hospice or palliative care, you have many resources. Doing an Internet search will give you some places to start. You can also ask your care team or people you meet in your support groups. Insurance covers the costs, and so does Medicare. (*Hospice Foundation* has a guide to get you started, https://hospicefoundation.org/End-of-Life-Support-and-Resources/Coping-with-Terminal-Illness/How-to-Access-Care.) The first step is talking with your loved ones, then talking to your health care providers. You have agency here to initiate these steps and take care of your needs.

Wills and Trusts

Again, as with many sources of support, an Internet search will turn up many options. One called *Freewill* (https://www.freewill.com) allows you to create a simple document for free.

Chapter Notes

Chapter 1

1. This is a reference to the *Bodhisattva's Four Methods of Guidance* Fascicle 46, contained in *Master Dogen's Shobo Genzo* (Tanahashi, 2013).

2. See Adorable (1971) for a review of emptiness and humanity.

Chapter 2

1. "The Sūtra of the Wheel of Dharma contains the Buddha's teaching to his five former spiritual companions on the four truths that he had discovered as part of his awakening: (1) suffering, (2) the origin of suffering, (3) the cessation of suffering, and (4) the path leading to the cessation of suffering. According to all the Buddhist traditions, this is the first teaching the Buddha gave to explain his awakened insight to others." See 84000: Translating the Words of the Buddha (2018), https://read.84000.co/translation/toh337.html#summary

2. Kyabgon (2015) has a very balanced discussion of this concept of co-dependent arising.

3. Marvin Gaye, "Inner City Blues (Make Me Wanna Holler)", YouTube.

Chapter 3

1. This bowing reenacts a bow as was done by one of the earlier followers of the Buddha, to ensure his feet would avoid stepping in a puddle (Lopez, 2013).

2. Dharmadhatu is the location of ultimate reality, where we live though we're unaware of it generally. Before our realization we are turned by it, rather than turning it. Knowing that we can instead turn a sutra, doing so removes us from the role of being acted on like a puppet. Instead, we use the time and encounters we have as we live to "actualize the fundamental point," as explained by Eihei Dogan. See Tanahashi (2013) or other translations of the Shobo Genzo fascicle, Actualizing the Fundamental Point.

3. This is a reference to the poem *The Song of the Jeweled Mirror Samadhi*, which is telling us about the Great Opportunity we have to become attentive and practice realization now in this life, https://www.sfzc.org/files/daily_sutras_Song_of_the_Jewel_Mirror_Samadhi.

Chapter 4

1. These payments influence doctors' prescribing decisions. "Sixty-seven percent of doctors received some kind of payment from 2015 to 2017. And in specialized areas—including oncology, urology and orthopedic surgery—that percentage jumped to more than 80%, according to researchers at Memorial Sloan Kettering Cancer Center in work funded by the National Cancer Institute. Physicians who receive money from a given company are more likely to prescribe that company's drug instead of other treatment options." More than $2 billion a year is paid by pharma companies to doctors. See https://

www.fiercepharma.com/marketing/more-money-more-prescriptions.

2. This "miracle" is explained in Eihei Dogan's Fascicle 26, *Miracles* (Tanahashi, 2013, p. 287). That is to say, it is natural to see this kind of outcome.

Chapter 5

1. Please visit https://www.healthcare.gov/get-coverage if you have low or no income. You must read carefully. Also know that the application process may be difficult, it's different in each state, and you may have to provide information initially and on an ongoing basis. You may feel sad as you go through the process. Zazen and Dance Practice help you set aside your ego and judgments. Please press forward so you can see the path before you.

2. "Recent studies have shown that chronic stress can induce tumorigenesis and promote cancer development. ... Chronic stress is heavily implicated in causing ill health, and today it is considered to encompass occupational stress as well as unusual adversities. Its potential negative effects include not only insomnia, gastrointestinal disorders, anxiety, and depression, but also an increased risk of cardiovascular disease, mental illness, and cancer" (Dai et al., 2020).

3. Eating foods that don't cause inflammation is critical to the reduction of diseases. Visit https://www.hopkinsmedicine.org/health/wellness-and-prevention/anti-inflammatory-diet for more details. It may take a minute to load this page.

Chapter 6

1. "What Happens If You Die Without a Will?" A. Hollyn Scott, Esq. at FindLaw (https://www.findlaw.com/forms/resources/estate-planning/last-will-and-testament/what-happens-if-i-die-without-a-will.html, 2024). This article has a good deal of information about the particulars of what happens without a will and trust. The details are a bit beyond the scope of this book.

2. This Internet site may be able to assist you. However, you'll need to provide your online credentials and such. https://www.freewill.com. Please know that this is only one; many others are out there.

3. See this U.S. government website hosted by the Federal Trade Commission for Consumer Advice, "Debts and Deceased Relatives": https://consumer.ftc.gov/articles/debts-and-deceased-relatives#whoisresponsible.

Bibliography

Acevedo-Garcia, D., Noelke, C., McArdle, N., Sofer, N., Hardy, E. F., Weiner, M., ... Reece, J. (2020). Racial and ethnic inequities in children's neighborhoods: Evidence from the New Child Opportunity Index 2.0. *Health Affairs, 39*(10), 1693–1701.

Adorable, V. H. (1971). The Zen concept of emptiness. *Asian Studies, 9*(1), 37–54. https://www.asj.upd.edu.ph/mediabox/archive/ASJ-09-01-1971/adorable-zen-concept-emptiness.pdf.

American Cancer Society. (n.d.). *Cancer Disparities in the Black Community.* https://www.cancer.org/about-us/what-we-do/health-equity/cancer-disparities-in-the-black-community.html.

American Cancer Society. (2019). *Cancer Facts & Figures for African Americans 2019–2021.* Atlanta, GA: American Cancer Society.

Anderson, R. (2001). *Being Upright: Zen Meditation and the Bodhisattva Precepts.* Berkeley, CA: Rodmell Press.

Anderson, R. (2012). *The Third Turning of the Wheel: Wisdom of the Samdhinirmocana Sutra.* Boulder, CO: Shambhala.

Avlijas, T., Squires, J. E., Lalonde, M., & Beckman, C. (2023). A concept analysis of the patient experience. *Patient Expérience Journal, 10*(1), 15–63. doi:10.35680/2372-0247.1439.

Ayhan, C. H.B., Bilgin, H., Uluman, O.T., Sukut, O., Yilmaz, S., & Buzlu, S. (2020). A systematic review of the discrimination against sexual and gender minority in health care settings. *International Journal of Health Services, 50*(1), 44–61. doi:10.1177/0020731419885093.

Baker, N. M. (2023). *Opening to Oneness: A Practical and Philosophical Guide to the Zen Precepts.* Boulder, CO: Shambhala.

Baraz, J., & Alexander, S. (2012). *Awakening Joy: 10 Steps to Happiness.* Berkeley, CA: Parallax Press.

Besser, L. (2021). *Dead white man's clothes.* ABC.Net.au. https://www.abc.net.au/news/2021-08-12/fast-fashion-turning-parts-ghana-into-toxic-landfill/100358702

Birmingham, S. (2024). *Certain People, America's Black Elite.* New York: Open Road Media.

Bitsko, R. H., Claussen, A. H., Lichstein, J., Black, L. I., Jones, S. E., Danielson, M. L., – Ghandour, R. M. (2022). Mental health surveillance among children—United States, 2013–2019. *Morbidity and Mortality Weekly Report Suppl. 71*(2), 1–42. DOI:http://dx.doi.org/10.15585/mmwr.su7102a1.

Brown, E. E. (2011). *The Complete Tassajara Cookbook: Recipes, Techniques, and Reflections from the Famed Zen Kitchen.* Boulder, CO: Shambhala.

Buddhism in America Timeline. Historical Development of Buddhism. Virginia Commonwealth University. https://tinyurl.com/39r4tst5, accessed August 23, 2024.

Bibliography

Chatzopoulos, G. S., Jiang, Z., Marka, N., & Wolff, L. F. (2024). Periodontal disease, tooth loss, and systemic conditions: An exploratory study. *International Dental Journal, 74*(2), 207–215. https://doi.org/10.1016/j.identj.2023.08.002.

Chinn, J. J., Martin. I. K., & Redmond, N. (2021). Health equity among black women in the United States. *Journal of Women's Health, 30*(2), 212–219. https://doi.org/10.1089/jwh.2020.8868

Cho, B., Han, Y., Lian, M., Colditz, G. A., Weber, J. D., Ma, C., & Liu, Y. (2021). Evaluation of racial/ethnic differences in treatment and mortality among women with triple-negative breast cancer. *JAMA Oncology, 7*(7), 1016–1023. doi:10.1001/jamaoncol.2021.1254.

Christian, T. A. (2022, February 16). Black Americans leave trillions in limbo without a will. *Ebony Magazine*, https://www.ebony.com/black-americans-leave-trillions-in-limbo-without-a-will.

Ch'ung-hsien. (2006) *The Blue Cliff Record*, trans. T. Cleary. Moraga, CA: BDK America.

Cruz, E. I. da S., Cruz, A. H. da S., Marques, R. A. S., Santos R. da S., & Reis, A. A. da S. (2022). The use of non-pharmacological adjuvant therapies for cancer pain: A narrative review in the context of dance. *Research, Society and Development, 11*(1), e30411124771, doi.org/10.33448/rsd-v11i1.24771.

Dai, S., Mo, Y., Wang, Y., Xiang, B., Liao, Q., Zhou M., ... Zeng, Z. (2020). Chronic stress promotes cancer development. *Frontiers in Oncology, 10*, 1492. https://doi.org/10.3389/fonc.2020.01492.

Dan Tao, D., Awan-Scully, R., Ash, G. I., Pei, Z., Gu, Y., Gao, Y., ... Baker, J. S. (2023). The effectiveness of dance movement interventions for older adults with mild cognitive impairment, Alzheimer's disease, and dementia: A systematic scoping review and meta-analysis. *Ageing Research Reviews, 92*, 102120. doi.org/10.1016/j.arr.2023.102120.

Davis, B. W. (2022). *Zen Pathways An Introduction to the Philosophy and Practice of Zen Buddhism*. New York: Oxford University Press.

Derman, B. A., Jasielec, J., Langerman, S. S., Zhang, W., Jakubowiak, A. J., & Chiu, B. C-H. (2000). Racial differences in treatment and outcomes in multiple myeloma: A Multiple Myeloma Research Foundation Analysis. *Blood Cancer Journal, 10*(80). doi.org/10.1038/s41408-020-00347-6.

Donaldson, M. S. (2004). Nutrition and cancer: A review of the evidence for an anti-cancer diet. *Nutrition Journal, 3*(19). doi:10.1186/1475-2891-3-19

Dussel, E. (1995). *The Invention of the Americas: Eclipse of "the Other" and the Myth of Modernity*. New York: Continuum. http://biblioteca.clacso.edu.ar/ar/libros/dussel/1492in/1492in.html.

Easwaran, E. (1993). *Meditation: A Simple Eight-Point Program for Translating Spiritual Ideals into Daily Life*. Tomales, CA: Nilgiri Press.

Edell, J. A., Stewart, D., and Hecker, S., eds. (1988). *Nonverbal Effects in Ads: A Review and Synthesis. in Nonverbal Communication in Advertising*. New York: Lexington Books.

84000: Translating the Words of the Buddha. (2018). *The Sūtra of the Wheel of Dharma*, trans. by the Dharmachakra Translation Committee. https://read.84000.co/translation/toh337.html#summary

Ewen, S. (1976). *Captains of Consciousness; Advertising and the Social Roots of the Consumer*. New York: McGraw-Hill.

Farmer, B. (2022, January 10). *Black-Owned Hospice Seeks to Bring Greater Ease in Dying to Black Families*. Nashville Public Radio. https://kffhealthnews.org/news/article/black-owned-hospice-end-of-life-care-disparities.

Bibliography

Gallagher. S. (2006). *How the Body Shapes the Mind.* New York: Oxford University Press.

Gavidia, M. (2023, January 11). *Spotlighting Health Disparities for Black Americans With Multiple Myeloma and Potential Solutions.* AJMC. https://www.ajmc.com/view/spotlighting-health-disparities-for-black-americans-with-multiple-myeloma-and-potential-solutions.

Gawande, A. (2014). *Being Mortal: Medicine and What Matters in the End.* New York: Metropolitan Books.

Geiger, H. J. (2003). Racial and ethnic disparities in diagnosis and treatment: A review of the evidence and a consideration of causes. In *Unequal Treatment: Confronting Racial and Ethnic Disparities in Health Care,* ed. B. D. Smedley, A. Y. Stith, and A. R. Nelson, Institute of Medicine, (US) Committee on Understanding and Eliminating Racial and Ethnic Disparities in Health Care. Washington, DC: National Academies Press. www.ncbi.nlm.nih.gov/books/NBK220337.

Gomes, N., Cochet, S., & Guyon, A. (2021). Dance and embodiment: Therapeutic benefits on body-mind health. *Journal of Interdisciplinary Methodologies and Issues in Science,* Methods to Assess the Effects of Sensory Stimulations on Wellness, 9. 10.18713/JIMIS-02072021-9-4.

Gordon, J. (2020, September 22). *Addressing the Crisis of Black Youth Suicide.* Director's Message, National Institute of Mental Health. https://www.nimh.nih.gov/about/director/messages/2020/addressing-the-crisis-of-black-youth-suicide

Hanh, T. N. (1999). *The Heart of the Buddha's Teaching: Transforming Suffering into Peace, Joy, and Liberation.* New York: Harmony.

Hanh, T. N. (2002). *Anger: Wisdom for Cooling the Flames.* New York: Riverhead Books.

Hanna, J. L. (1987). *To Dance Is Human; A Theory of Nonverbal Communication.* Chicago: University of Chicago Press.

Hensley, L. (2021, February 5). Dying at home may improve patient satisfaction surrounding end-of-life care. *Verywell Health News.* https://www.verywellhealth.com/palliative-care-should-consider-patients-preferences-5104799.

Houseal, J. (2020 August 8). *Three Aspects of Buddhist Dance.* BDG. https://www.buddhistdoor.net/features/three-aspects-of-buddhist-dance.

Imbesi, S., Allegra, A., Calapi, G., Musolino, C. & Gangemi, S. (2015). Cutaneous adverse reactions to lenalidomide. *Allergologia et Immunopathologica, 43*(1), 88–91. DOI:10.1016/j.aller.2013.07.005.

Ingini, M. (2023, August 21). 10 Concerning fast fashion waste statistics. *Global Commons,* Earth.Org. https://earth.org/statistics-about-fast-fashion-waste/#:~:text=3.,landfills%20on%20a%20yearly%20basis

Janssens, R., Long, T., Vallejo, A., Galinsky, J., Plate, A., Morgan, K., ... Huys, I. (2021). Patient preferences for multiple myeloma treatments: A multinational qualitative study. *Frontiers in Medicine, 8,* 686165, doi:10.3389/fmed.2021.686165.

Johns Hopkins Medicine. (n.d.). *Anti Inflammatory Diet.* https://www.hopkinsmedicine.org/health/wellness-and-prevention/anti-inflammatory-diet

Kanapuru, B. (2022). Analysis of racial and ethnic disparities in multiple myeloma US FDA drug approval trials. *Blood Advances, 6*(6), 1684–169. doi:10.1182/bloodadvances.2021005482

Kim, H.-J. (2000). *Eihei Dogen: Mystical Realist,* rev. ed. Somerville, MA: Wisdom Publications.

Klahr, S. (2020, December 3). *Pharma payments to physicians still deliver a big 'return on investment' in prescription growth, study finds.* https://www.fiercepharma.com/marketing/more-money-more-prescriptions

Kumar, K. S., Srinivasan, T. M., Ilavarasu, J., Mondal, B., & Nagendra, H. R. (2018).

Bibliography

Classification of electrophotonic images of yogic practice of mudra through neural networks. *International Journal of Yoga, 11*(2), 152–156. https://www.ncbi.nlm.nih.gov/pmc/articles/PMC5934951.

Kusunoki, R. K. (2002). The origin of Obon. *Wheel of the Sangha, Newsletter, 42*(7), 1.

Kwong, J. R. (2022). Illuminate your true self. *Tricycle*, Spring.

Kyabgon, T. (2015). *Karma: What It Is, What It Isn't, Why It Matters.* Boulder, CO: Shambhala.

Lateef, H., Gale, A., Jellesma, F., & Borgstrom, E. (2024). "The belief to aspire": The association between Afrocentric values in the educational and career aspirations of young black males. *Urban Review, 56*, 19–34. https://doi.org/10.1007/s11256-023-00680-7.

Levy, F. J. (1995). *Dance and Other Expressive Art Therapies: When Words Are Not Enough.* New York: Routledge.

Lopez, D. S., Jr. (2009). *The Story of Buddhism: A Concise Guide to Its History & Teachings.* New York: HarperOne.

Lopez, D. S., Jr. (2013) *From Stone to Flesh: A Short History of the Buddha.* Chicago: Chicago University Press.

Manuel, Z. E. (2022, September 18). *All Experience Is Perceived by Mind.* San Francisco Zen Center, Green Gulch Farm, Dharma Talk. https://www.sfzc.org/teachings/dharma-talks/all-experience-perceived-mind-0

Mark, J. J. (2020, September 28). The dates of the Buddha. *World History Encyclopedia.*. https://www.worldhistory.org/article/493/the-dates-of-the-buddha.

Mateos, M.-V., Weisel, K., De Stefano, V., Goldschmidt, H., Delforge, M., Mohty, M., ... Moreau, P. (2022). LocoMMotion: A prospective, non-interventional, multinational study of real-life current standards of care in patients with relapsed and/or refractory multiple myeloma. *Leukemia, 36*, 1371–1376. doi.org/10.1038/s41375-022-01531-2.

McCracken, G. D. (1986). Culture and consumption: A theoretical account of the structure and movement of the cultural meaning of consumer goods. *Journal of Consumer Research, 13*(1), 71–84.

Medina-Martínez, J., Saus-Ortegs, C., Sánchez-Lorente, M. M., Sosa-Palanca, E. M., García-Martinez, P., & Mármol-López, M. I. (2021). Health inequities in LGBT people and nursing interventions to reduce them: A systematic review. *International Journal of Environmental Research and Public Health, 18*(22), 11801. https://doi.org/10.3390/ijerph182211801.

Melby, C., Mosendz, P., & Buhayar, N. (2024, July 24). The miseducation of America's nurse practitioners. *Bloomberg Businessweek.* https://www.bloomberg.com/news/features/2024-07-24/is-the-nurse-practitioner-job-boom-putting-us-health-care-at-risk?embedded-checkout=true.

Mitchell, A. P., Truvedi, N. U., Gennarelli, R. L., Chimonas, S., Tabatabai, S. M., Goldberg, J., ... Korentstein, D. (2021). Are financial payments from the pharmaceutical industry associated with physician prescribing? A systematic review. *Annals of Internal Medicine, 174*(3), 353–361. doi:10.7326/M20-5665.

Nagarjuna, A., & B. Dharmamitra (trans.). (2009). *Nagarjuna on the Six Perfections.* Seattle, WA: Kalavinka Press.

Nishimura, K. K., Barlogie, B., van Rhee, F., Zangari, M., Walker, B. A., Rosenthal, A., ... Morgan, G. J. (2020). Long-term outcomes after autologous stem cell transplantation for multiple myeloma. *Blood Advances, 4*(2), 422–431. doi.org/10.1182/bloodadvances.2019000524.

Nuriddin, A., Mooney, G., & White, A. I. R. (2020). Reckoning with histories of medical racism and violence in the USA. *Lancet, 396*(10256), 949–951. doi:https://doi.org/10.1016/S0140-6736(20)32032-8.

Bibliography

Paterick, T. J., Carson, G. V., Allen, M. C., & Paterick, T. E. (2008). Medical informed consent: General considerations for physicians. *Mayo Clinic Proceedings, 83*(3), 313–319. doi:https://doi.org/10.4065/83.3.313.

Perez-Kempner, L. (2019, September 14). What is revlimid? *Medical News Today.* www.medicalnewstoday.com/articles/326466#_noHeaderPrefixedContent.

Reynolds, F. E., et al. (2024). Buddhism. *Encyclopedia Britannica.* https://www.britannica.com/topic/Buddhism.

Ruiz-Muelle, A., & López-Rodríguez, M. M. (2019). Dance for people with Alzheimer's disease: A systematic review. *Current Alzheimer Research, 16*(10), 919–933. doi:doi.org/10.2174/1567205016666190725151614.

Rutschman-Byler, J. M. (2009). *Two Shores of Zen: An American Monk's Japan.* Lulu.com.

Sausser, L. (2024, July 2). Med schools face a new obstacle in the push to train more Black doctors. *SHOTS Health News*, NPR.

Sayed, A., Ross, J. S., & Mandrola, J. (2024). Industry payments to US physicians by specialty and product type. *JAMA, 331*(15), 1325–1327. doi:10.1001/jama.2024.1989.

Scott, A. H. (2024). *What happens if you die without a will?* FindLaw. https://tinyurl.com/dy4zrers.

Shunryu, S. R. (2009). *Not Always So: Practicing the True Spirit of Zen.* New York: HarperOne.

Shunryu, S. R. (2011). *Zen Mind, Beginner's Mind: Informal Talks on Zen Meditation and Practice.* Boulder, CO: Shambhala.

Sturm, I., Baak, J., Storek, B., Traore, A., & Thuss-Patience, P. (2014). Effect of dance on cancer-related fatigue and quality of life. *Supportive Care in Cancer, 22*, 2241–2249. doi.org/10.1007/s00520-014-2181-8.

Swami, O. (2024). *Kinhin and Sleep Meditation: Embracing Awareness in Movement.* https://tinyurl.com/3hsxaj7v

Tanahashi, K., editor (2013). *Treasury of the True Dharma Eye: Zen Master Dogen's Shobo Genzo.* Boulder, CO: Shambhala.

Tao, Dan, et al. (2023). The effectiveness of dance movement interventions for older adults with mild cognitive impairment, alzheimer's disease, and dementia: A systematic scoping review and meta-analysis. *Ageing Research Reviews* 92. doi.org/10.1016/j.arr.2023.102120.

Taylor, J. K. (2021). Structural racism and maternal health among Black women. *Journal of Law, Medicine & Ethics, 48*(3), 506–517. https://doi.org/10.1177/1073110520958875.

Thiagarajan, P., & Mokthar, M. K. (2022). Self-rehabilitation through dance: An Ethnographic Study on Candy Girls Breast Cancer Survivor Group in Kuala Lumpur, Malaysia. *Kajian Malaysia, 40*(1), 39–58. doi.org/10.21315/km2022.40.1.3.

Uchiyama, K. R. (2004). *Opening the Hand of Thought: Foundations of Zen Buddhist Practice,* Somerville, MA: Wisdom Publications.

Walter, C. S. (2012). Dance in advertising: The silent persuader. *Advertising & Society Review, 13*(3). https://muse.jhu.edu/pub/21/article/491082.

Walter, C. S. (2015). *Dance, Consumerism, and Spirituality.* London: Palgrave.

Walter, C. S. (2020). *Sacred Dance Meditations: 365 Globally Inspired Movement Practices Enhancing Awakening, Clarity, and Connection.* Berkeley, CA: North Atlantic Books.

Weis, J., Troitzsch, A., & Dresch, C. (2022). Dance theatre as a form of dance movement psychotherapy for male cancer survivors. *Body, Movement and Dance in Psychotherapy, 17*(3), 200–217. doi:10.1080/17432979.2021.1962406.

Weitsman, S. M. (2008). *Dharma talk on birth and death.* Chapel Hill Zen Center. https://www.chzc.org/mel27.htm

Bibliography

Wikipedia. (n.d.). *Juneteenth*. https://en.wikipedia.org/wiki/Juneteent .

Wikipedia. (n.d.). *Timeline of Zen Buddhism in the United States*. https://en.wikipedia.org/wiki/Timeline_of_Zen_Buddhism_in_the_United_States.

Williams, J. M., Wilson. S. K., & Bergeson, C. (2020). Health implications of incarceration and reentry on returning citizens: A qualitative examination of Black men's experiences in a northeastern city. *American Journal of Men's Health, 14*(4). doi:10.1177/1557988320937211.

Woodson, C. G. (1999). *The Mis-Education of the Negro.* Originally published 1933. Swanee, GA: 12th Media Services,.

Worthington, R. (2024, February 5). *Unique Caregiving Challenges the Black Community Is Navigating and What Can Help.* https://www.care.com/c/caregiving-challenges-faced-by-black-community.

Yearby, R., Clark, B., and Figueroa, J. F. (2022). Structural racism in historical and modern US health care policy. *Health Affairs, 41*(2). https://doi.org/10.1377/hlthaff.2021.01466.

Zarei, E., Ghaffari, A., Nikoobar, A., Bastami, S., & Hamdghaddari, H. (2022). Interaction between physicians and the pharmaceutical industry: A scoping review for developing a policy brief. *Frontiers in Public Health, 10.* doi:10.3389/fpubh.2022.1072708.

Index

Index